100 Questions & Answers About Influenza

Delthia Ricks, MA, MS
Medical Writer, *Newsday*

Foreword by
Marc Siegel, MD
Associate Professor
New York University
New York, NY
FOX News contributor

JONES AND BARTLETT PUBLISHERS
Sudbury, Massachusetts
BOSTON   TORONTO   LONDON   SINGAPORE

World Headquarters

Jones and Bartlett Publishers
40 Tall Pine Drive
Sudbury, MA 01776
978-443-5000
info@jbpub.com
www.jbpub.com

Jones and Bartlett Publishers
Canada
6339 Ormindale Way
Mississauga, Ontario L5V 1J2
Canada

Jones and Bartlett Publishers
International
Barb House, Barb Mews
London W6 7PA
United Kingdom

Jones and Bartlett's books and products are available through most bookstores and online booksellers. To contact Jones and Bartlett Publishers directly, call 800-832-0034, fax 978-443-8000, or visit our Web site, www.jbpub.com.

Substantial discounts on bulk quantities of Jones and Bartlett's publications are available to corporations, professional associations, and other qualified organizations. For details and specific discount information, contact the special sales department at Jones and Bartlett via the above contact information or send an email to specialsales@jbpub.com.

The authors, editor, and publisher have made every effort to provide accurate information. However, they are not responsible for errors, omissions, or for any outcomes related to the use of the contents of this book and take no responsibility for the use of the products and procedures described. Treatments and side effects described in this book may not be applicable to all people; likewise, some people may require a dose or experience a side effect that is not described herein. Drugs and medical devices are discussed that may have limited availability controlled by the Food and Drug Administration (FDA) for use only in a research study or clinical trial. Research, clinical practice, and government regulations often change the accepted standard in this field. When consideration is being given to use of any drug in the clinical setting, the healthcare provider or reader is responsible for determining FDA status of the drug, reading the package insert, and reviewing prescribing information for the most up-to-date recommendations on dose, precautions, and contraindications, and determining the appropriate usage for the product. This is especially important in the case of drugs that are new or seldom used.

Production Credits

Executive Publisher: Christopher Davis
Associate Editor: Kathy Richardson
Senior Editorial Assistant: Jessica Acox
Production Director: Amy Rose
Production Editor: Daniel Stone
Marketing Manager: Ilana Goddess

V.P. of Manufacturing and Inventory Control:
  Therese Connell
Composition: Shawn Girsberger
Printing and Binding: Malloy, Inc.
Cover Printing: Malloy, Inc.

Cover Credits

Cover Design: Kristin E. Parker
Top Photo: Courtesy of National Archives, photo no. 165-WW-269B-25; Bottom Left Photo: Courtesy of the Centers for Disease Control and Prevention; Bottom Right Photo: © David Hughes/Dreamstime.com.

Library of Congress Cataloging-in-Publication Data

Ricks, Delthia.
  100 questions and answers about influenza / Delthia Ricks.
    p. cm.
  Includes bibliographical references and index.
  ISBN-13: 978-0-7637-4501-1
  ISBN-10: 0-7637-4501-4
  1. Influenza--Miscellanea. 2. Influenza viruses--Miscellanea. 3. Influenza--Popular works. 4. Influenza viruses--Popular works. I. Title. II. Title: One hundred questions and answers about influenza.
  RC150.R46 2009
  616.2'03--dc22

                        2008028727

6048

Printed in the United States of America
12 11 10 09 08   10 9 8 7 6 5 4 3 2 1

For my daughters,

Kimberly and Kourtney

CONTENTS

Contents

Recently, the term "plain talk" has lost its positive context, at least in political circles. But when I use this term to describe Delthia Ricks, longtime topflight health reporter for *Newsday*, I intend the term in the most positive of ways. Influenza may be the most misunderstood and slippery of all current health topics, and Ricks, in this clear, informative, and well-researched book, gives us the "plain talk" on flu that we—as a society frequently riddled with health scares—most sorely need.

It used to be that flu was underappreciated. Health pundits and journalists alike hauled it out as our yearly example of a massive killer that ran below the radar because it just wasn't sexy. Back in the 1960s in Japan, the government mandated flu vaccines for all children for most of the next 25 years. Since kids are among the biggest spreaders of flu (schools are viral swamps), this "experiment" led to a decrease of deaths from all causes of over a million people.

But this incredible societal example of the effects of influenza was largely ignored in the United States. Back in the day when flu was not yet provoking fear, yet was killing 36,000 Americans every year and hospitalizing hundreds of thousands, flu was poorly understood. It still is. The influenza virus is pleomorphic, meaning it mutates frequently and changes its infectivity. Influenza also wears down the immune system and leads to life threatening illness from other causes, including, though not limited to pneumonia, sinusitis, otitis, heart attacks, and sepsis.

Ricks explains all this, and more importantly, she explains the flu, flu vaccines, and flu pandemics, and in this explaining, she reduces our flu fears. This is crucial. Fear comes from the unknown. Information is the treatment for fear. But not just any information. For information to be a truly effective antidote for worry it must be accurate and properly contexted. Ricks is an expert at providing context.

Four years ago, the bar was raised much higher regarding the need for a proper and persuasive explanation of flu. In late 2005, the whole conversation surrounding flu suddenly changed. This tricky and potentially deadly bug suddenly went from being a "ho-hum" killer, as I termed it then, to a sinister, mystery killer, with constant references and allusions to the 1918 blue death, the third greatest plague in the history of mankind.

Close followers of the news remember exactly why this happened. Speculative reports and speculating reporters pointed to a highly pathogenic bird flu known as H5N1 as the next "blue death." The blurring of distinctions between the 1918 scourge, the yearly flu, and a potential new bird flu pandemic led to a growing fear of flu that replaced the prior ignorance about this virus.

Lost in this growing media-fueled panic (a 2006 AP/IPSOS poll found that 35% of Americans believed that either they or a relative was going to be infected by H5N1 bird flu) were the scientific facts: (1) H5N1, though it has killed millions of birds, has only killed a few hundred people, and is not easily passed from human to human; (2) the last three human pandemics were NOT caused by highly pathogenic H5 bird viruses like H5N1 that transformed into killer human viruses; they were cause by H1, H2, and H3 viruses; and (3) though it is believed that the 1918 massive pandemic was caused by a bird-like virus mutating into a form that killed millions of humans, it is unclear exactly how that happened or that the conditions are somehow parallel with H5N1.

In this careful book, Ricks distinguishes between the yearly flu strains, which are often distant descendants of the 1918 flu to which we now have developed significant immunity, and the current bird flu, which is a remote risk. She writes about the best ways to prepare for the flu, as well as how to prevent its spread. She utilizes proper information to reduce fear in the best sense. In fact, it is the human tendency to blur current reality with worst case potential that has caused us to both under-appreciate and overreact to the flu. Ricks helps us learn to distinguish.

She brings up the dramatic example of the 1976 swine flu fiasco to demonstrate what happens when we overreact in *anticipation* of a worst case scenario. In 1976, a massive inoculation campaign to 40 million people of a hastily prepared swine flu vaccine in response to an imagined threat from a pig flu (the prevailing theory of the time was that pigs served as mixing vessels for emerging pandemic strains) appears to have led to close to 1,000 cases of ascending paralysis (Guillain-Barre Syndrome) in those who received the vaccine. This is a mistake we should learn from and not make again. But the hysterical concerns about H5N1 in 2006 suggest that we haven't learned enough.

Ricks does far more than bring up historical and cultural examples to simultaneously warn us as well as prepare us. She examines the risks of the yearly flu, describes how it evolves and is tracked, and explains how vaccines are currently prepared. Ricks describes both the limitations and the advantages of the current flu vaccine, citing current research. She correctly points out that available technology could be utilized to upgrade how we make vaccines by growing them in mammalian cells, rather than in chicken eggs (which are often killed by the virus we are breeding). Channeling our resources towards vaccine upgrades using state-of-the art technology would provide the ability to make vaccines far more rapidly than the current 9 months it takes to make a usable batch. This would give us the ability to *react* to an emerging strain rather than have to nervously *anticipate* one.

The nuts and bolts of flu are important to everyone, not just physicians. Doctors and patients can work together to slow the spread and to contain it when it is in our midst. Flu weakens and kills, but it can also be controlled. Ricks provides the information we need to react practically to the flu. More than that, she provides the kind of sober approach we can use to approach all our infectious diseases.

This book is written in a question and answer format that anticipates your questions and then answers them. It is written by a consummate writer and careful journalist, a rare combination these days. Ricks is informative without being inflammatory, definitive about a scary virus without being scary.

Marc Siegel, MD

Dr. Siegel is an internist and an associate professor of medicine at New York University's School of Medicine. He is also the author of *False Alarm: The Truth About the Epidemic of Fear.* He is also a FOX News Medical Contributor.

On the front porch that overlooked two Pride-of-China trees, my grandfather, whose throne was a high-backed rocker, would reminisce about his youth. He was a riveting storyteller. His words were so steeped in imagery that listeners could be quickly transported backward in time, seeing what he saw as a child: the so called "packing houses" of Omaha where cattle were slaughtered and butchered into steaks. Another sharp image was the banks of the Big Muddy, the Missouri River, which cuts a turbulent swath through Nebraska.

Through that imagery rose a series of stories about the early 20th century, which from his view of the period seemed to be a world filled with horses, dust and medical conditions that I felt never could cause affliction in a modern, technologically driven time.

Or could these illnesses strike again?

One of his most repeated stories was about "the grippe," a disease that had a strange name and unquestionably chilling consequences. He told of having to wear a white gauze mask, of seeing men, women and children whom he knew being carried from their homes as corpses. Schools and businesses were closed. Church services were banned. And he often spoke of restrictions imposed by a quickly organized quarantine. I am almost certain that I must have been around the age of 8 when that word became part of my vocabulary, although I must admit, I didn't fully understand its meaning— nor the strange disease he called the grippe.

Years would pass before I realized that I had been transported to 1918 and to the quickly organized ground war against a horrific influenza strain. Some call it the Spanish Flu. More recent authors have characterized it as the *Devil's Flu* and *The Great Influenza*.

Thoughts of "the grippe" crystallized for me in 1989 when I caught the flu—a bout so serious, I developed pneumonia.

At the time, I was working as a science writer for UPI, United Press International in Los Angeles, where I frequently wrote about influenza and the ever-changing genetic character of flu viruses. As someone who also holds a graduate degree in biology, I was well aware—and often reported—that flu shots must be administered on an annual basis because of the rapid mutation rate of influenza viruses. The shot you receive this year will not protect you next year because the viruses in circulation have altered their genetic makeup.

But what makes people not practice what they preach?

Young and healthy, I blithely thought—somewhere in the recesses of my mind—that flu shots were for old people and the sickly, despite what I was dispensing as important health information for everybody else.

Although I am not 100 percent certain, I believe the virus I caught in January of 1989 must have been the relatively rare Hong Kong B strain, which was causing epidemics throughout the United States in the 1988-89 flu season. The strain rose again in 2002 to cause a wave of flu infections across the country.

At peak flu season the year I caught the flu, UPI was the perfect incubator for influenza's spread. The office, in an old brick building in downtown Los Angeles, was small, cramped, and rarely cleaned. The cash-strapped owners could not afford to buy enough computers, so people shared equipment in a place that was open around the clock. Smoking was allowed and the smokers would fill the place with a cloud so thick that a smog-like haze hung permanently just below ceiling height. Coughers and sneezers simply didn't care. Keyboards were grimy. Who knows what could have been cultured from them? And, when Bob, the chain-smoking, foul-mouthed managing editor happened to catch you spraying a keyboard with disinfectant he was certain to bark: "This ain't a damn hospital it's a newsroom. You're paid to punch those keys not clean 'em."

In retrospect, I suppose it should not have come as a surprise that when a "bug was going around," everyone invariably would catch it. Reporters seemed to be stricken one-by-one, until eventually virtually everyone in the office caught it. Even Bob was brought down—but he mustered enough strength to work while sick, something public health experts now strongly discourage.

I started coughing on a Friday night at home and fearing that I had a "bad cold," asked my husband, Tim, to take our two small daughters to my parents' home where they would not be exposed to whatever I had caught at work. By Saturday morning I could not lift my head from my pillow. My head throbbed as never before. To this day, the muscle aches remain indescribable. I spiked a fever that kept rising until it hit 103 degrees. Nothing made it go away. Days later when symptoms still hadn't abated and I was feeling worse, my husband insisted that I see our physician at Kaiser Permanente, the HMO.

Our doctor, a woman, who at the time was in her sixties, immediately recognized influenza symptoms and said she also wanted to test for pneumonia. As she was filling out laboratory forms, she said something that I hadn't heard in years. "Yes, I think you've got the old grippe. Do you know that term, the grippe?"

Did I know the term?

Is grass green? Is the sky not blue? Of course I knew it.

"Most people don't use that term much anymore," she said.

I explained that my grandfather who loved to tell stories about the past used that term all of the time in reference to the flu. But he also used it in discussions about a flu outbreak that required him to wear a mask.

"Spanish flu," the doctor said, facing me to explain her family's experience with a virus that killed 40 million people worldwide. Two of her uncles who had fought in France during WW I perished not as a result of the battle, but of the flu that arrived at the tail end of the war.

She assured me that I didn't have anything even remotely as grave as the Spanish flu, but that I would have to take it easy, certainly if, as she suspected, I also had pneumonia.

Scant as my knowledge was about the 1918 flu, my physician was impressed that I knew something about it. At the time, it was not discussed often, and several generations of physicians were practicing who didn't know much about the carnage the flu created. Then she said something I will never forget: "The flu is a very serious infection, especially when it has complications like yours. The flu still kills, you know."

My test came back positive for pneumonia, which lengthened my recovery, but at the same time prompted something more lasting. For essentially two decades I have ritualistically lined up for a flu shot. As a result of experiencing a complex bout of influenza, I now understand the importance of vaccination and why, even if others around me fail to be vaccinated, at least I won't be a link in the chain of transmission.

I have great respect for the flu's consequences and am fully cognizant that influenza is not a viral infection that can be taken lightly. I still have strong images from my grandfather's recollections as he witnessed a pandemic unfold before his eyes. He probably would be intrigued to learn that the virus at the heart of the 1918 grippe originated in birds, and then mutated into a globe-circling form easily transmissible among humans. He probably would be very concerned when told scientists today are closely monitoring another bird virus that could undergo a similar series of mutations and revive the specter of the 1918 influenza.

Delthia Ricks

PART ONE

Influenza 101

What is influenza? Isn't it really just a bad form of the common cold?

How are respiratory infections spread?

Are the stomach flu or the 24-hour 'flu bug' infections genuine influenza?

More . . .

influenza

A serious respiratory infection noteworthy for its rapid person-to-person spread. Influenza can have a limited impact on a community or it can spread rapidly throughout many communities as an epidemic.

Influenza is a virus that can be propelled at a rate nearing the speed of sound during the course of a single cough.

Centers for Disease Control and Prevention (CDC)

The leading U.S. government health agency that helps to prevent and control infectious and chronic diseases.

immune system

The cells, tissues, and organs that help body resist infection and disease by producing antibodies themselves to block the multiplication of the agent.

1. What is influenza? Isn't it really just a bad form of the common cold?

Influenza—the **flu**—is a highly contagious respiratory infection caused by a virus that can be propelled at a rate nearing the speed of sound during the course of a single cough. Scientists who have studied the act of coughing proved this in a sophisticated series of tests that examined the expulsion of secretions as they were forced from the respiratory tracts of flu sufferers. Without going into a lot of complicated calculations, a profusion of viruses is already in the air by the time you hear an infected person's cough. A single cough—or sneeze—can propel flu viruses 15 feet.

Although few people think about the physics involved in spreading the flu, virtually everybody has a flu story: how the infection knocked them out and sent them to bed for a week; or how they *cured* it with chicken soup or by sipping tea laced with lemon juice and honey. And why shouldn't such flu tales abound? The **Centers for Disease Control and Prevention (CDC)** estimates that influenza infects a staggering percentage of the U.S. population each flu season, which runs from late fall through early spring. The CDC finds that anywhere from 5% to 20% of the U.S. population catches the flu, which annually amounts to millions of feverish people who are coughing, aching, and sneezing from November through March. Within that short span each year, anywhere from 36,000 to 50,000 people die of flu complications, generally pneumonia. Globally, the death toll is 20 times to 30 times as high as that in the United States.

Influenza is caused by any of the viruses belonging to the complex groups that have been simply labeled A, B, and C. In Question 3, we explore in greater detail what these designations mean. Flu viruses are notorious for the speed with which they mutate, which means undergo genetic change, a characteristic that has allowed them for countless millennia to outfox the human **immune system** and invade cells of the respiratory tract.

Suffice it to say the flu definitely is not a nastier form of the **common cold.** Viruses also trigger the common cold, but the families to which flu and common cold viruses belong are only distantly related. Elsewhere in the book we explore the nature of viruses in more depth. For now, to fully understand influenza—what it is and what it isn't—you first may want to brush aside any myths harbored about this respiratory infection and lore about its treatment.

2. I've heard that chicken soup can cure the flu. Is that a myth?

Although some scientific studies have concluded that chicken soup may have medicinal value, there isn't a single substance afloat in the broth that possesses antiviral properties. Perhaps chicken soup acts as a comfort food at a time when you're feeling particularly awful, and the psychological boost it provides lifts your spirits. Some people have insisted that a shot of another kind of *spirits* has sent their bout with the flu into retreat. Vodka, whiskey, and rum all have been touted as 80-proof influenza cures. But homemade flu cures are products of an imprecise science. Cultural beliefs, family traditions, and a host of old wives' tales govern how people cope with the flu, primarily because it's a condition that has mostly been nursed at home. Hence, there may be more to the chicken soup cure than you might think: Soup helps provide hydration and nutrition, both of which are important during a viral illness, and especially influenza because fever depletes the body's fluid balance and appetite is suppressed during the illness.

You may be surprised to learn that fables about influenza seem to circulate as readily as flu viruses themselves, and physicians often remark with surprise that they are still dispelling notions about the flu, even now in the 21st century. You can't catch the flu by standing in the rain, wading through puddles, or sleeping in a drafty room. You can't catch the flu from a flu shot. And the common cold cannot worsen and transform into influenza.

common cold

A highly contagious, upper respiratory condition caused by any one of many types of viruses. The common cold is typified by nasal congestion, coughing, sneezing, sore throats, and, in some instances, temporarily losing the ability to taste foods or hear clearly.

Cultural beliefs, family traditions, and a host of old wives' tales govern how people cope with the flu, primarily because it's a condition that has mostly been nursed at home.

Influenza 101

strain

A genetic variant or subtype of a microorganism. The strain is determined by the genetic differences in proteins that make up the flu virus.

vaccine

A preparation consisting of a weakened or killed pathogen that stimulates the immune system to fend off infection by producing antibodies.

pandemic

A global outbreak of diseususes higher rates of sickness and death as occurred three times in the 20th century during major flu outbreaks that killed millions of people.

With that said, influenza and the common cold share several symptoms. So many, in fact, that even your doctor may not be able to discern a difference without ordering a special laboratory test to isolate an offending flu virus to confirm a case of influenza. Both the flu and the common cold affect the respiratory tract. Both are seasonal illnesses. Both make your nose run and head ache. But the flu is much more complex, and symptoms tend to be far more intense.

The flu can lead to pneumonia or secondary bacterial infections, complications that generally don't occur when you're affected by the common cold. Also, the flu can vary in the way it spreads through populations. A flu season can prove mild or moderate, or strains in circulation can lead to local outbreaks and nationwide epidemics. Virus-tracking scientists, as we shall learn in greater depth in Questions 6 and 21, conduct routine surveillance as influenza viruses circumnavigate the globe. By tracking circulating viruses in the Southern Hemisphere (where flu season occurs earlier in the year than in the Northern Hemisphere), public health officials know with some degree of certainty which **strains** are most likely to cause illnesses by the time the infections are being felt in northern latitudes. Identifying those strains early in the year helps public health officials make the most precise choice for the annual **vaccine**.

There is a darker side to influenza viruses, something that will never happen with the common cold. On some occasions a circulating strain of flu possesses a genetic makeup that is so foreign to human populations that it spawns a global **pandemic**. This form of influenza is rare, but it is the most feared. Pandemic flu strains circumvented the world in the last century in 1918, 1957, and 1968.

Yet, even with a reputation for circling the globe, many people consider influenza to be nothing more than a wintertime annoyance, something that arrives with other unavoidable seasonal nuisances: cold weather, bulkier clothing, and higher home heating bills. Television commercials also seem to have downgraded the importance of influenza by giving it second billing in so-called cold and flu season.

Anyone who has ever been seriously waylaid by influenza can tell you that the fever, the dry cough, aches, and chills are not symptoms to be taken lightly. As will be discussed in greater detail in Question 3, thousands of people are hospitalized annually for flu complications, and, as mentioned earlier, a significant number die as a result of the infection.

Despite such seriousness, a survey of more than a thousand U.S. adults conducted by the National Foundation for Infectious Diseases found that a significant proportion of Americans do not take wintertime flu seriously. Forty-three percent, the foundation found, do not believe the infection is serious enough to warrant vaccination. Another 38% didn't believe they were at risk of catching it, and 37% blithely said they were not concerned about spreading the flu to friends or family members. In summary, the results of the survey suggest that many Americans have grown complacent in their views about influenza.

3. What should I know about differences between the flu and the common cold?

The flu tends to come on suddenly accompanied by fever, headache, sore throat, and body aches. You cough and sneeze. Your eyes may become sensitive to light. You may be hot one moment but shivering the next. You are likely to feel so overwhelmed by fatigue—and just generally out of sorts—that it is difficult to pull yourself out of bed. The infection invades the respiratory tract—the nasal passages, throat, and lungs. The telltale symptoms can be mild, moderate, or severe. There are several noteworthy complications. The illness can leave some people vulnerable to pneumonia and secondary bacterial infections. The CDC estimates that so many people are sickened annually by influenza that about 200,000 people in the United States must be hospitalized. As mentioned in Question 1, the flu claims thousands of lives annually all over the world. Many of the infection's victims are infants or elderly who die of severe respiratory complications.

A flu infection also can prove problematic for people with respiratory conditions such as asthma or chronic obstructive pulmonary disease (COPD); or anyone who has a condition that severely suppresses immunity, such as HIV infection; or while on cancer chemotherapy. Because the flu can prove deadly, public health authorities have emphasized the importance of vaccination, especially for the very young and the very old and for those with immune-compromising conditions.

As for the common cold, symptoms mount much more slowly than do those marking the sudden, achy onset of the flu. Usually a runny nose is the first sign that a cold is taking hold. The infection tends to affect the upper respiratory tract: the nasal passages, **Eustachian tubes** (the narrow canals that link the middle ear to the throat), and the bronchial tree of the lungs. You may or may not feel miserable, depending on the severity of the infection. A cold can temporarily rob you of your sense of taste and ability to breathe easily. Your ears may seem clogged. You may have sniffles that progress to considerable nasal stuffiness. Congestion leads to a productive cough. Even without coughing or sniffling, those around you will know you're ailing with a cold because your voice sounds different.

Type A

Pathogen that belongs to the family of orthomyxoviruses. all three major pandemics in the 20th century and the major pandemic of 1889 were caused by Type A flu strains.

The key differences between influenza and the common cold are the pathogens that cause them. As mentioned in Question 1, flu viruses fall under three major groupings: A, B, and C, and within Type A there are noteworthy subtypes. Type A influenza not only is the most common of the trio, but the one to be taken very seriously because various strains have been associated with severe outbreaks and epidemics. A major feature of **Type A** flu viruses is their capacity to infect both humans and animals. Historically, it has been Type A viruses that have triggered globe-sweeping pandemics. Indeed, all of the strains that caused worldwide pandemics and unusually high mortality in the 20th century were Type A influenza viruses. **Avian influenza,** the type of flu now fueling a global pandemic in birds, is a Type A strain, known as H5N1. Labeling Type A subtypes with *H* and *N* along with very specific numbers is yet another way scientists further identify Type A viruses. The shorthand designations speak volumes about the virulence of a strain. The *H* stands for **hemagglutinin,** one of the proteins on the viral surface. *N* stands for **neuraminidase**, another major protein that flu viruses rely on to infect the cells of their **hosts.**

The annual flu vaccine generally provides protection against two subtypes of influenza A and one strain of Type B.

Type B viruses also are a cause of epidemics and are noteworthy for outbreaks worldwide—especially those that occur among children—moving in waves of infection that produce significant absenteeism in schools. Together, A and B are the types that produce illnesses significant enough to lead to hospitalization. Nevertheless, there still are several notable differences. Type A viruses can infect both humans and animals; Type B infects only people. The more limited range of hosts helps explain why influenza B viruses are not associated with pandemics. Scientists also know that Type B influenza tends to mutate at a slower pace compared with many Type A strains.

Generally speaking, influenza caused by Type B viruses is not as severe as illnesses caused by Type A strains, and Type B is not divided into subtypes. But that doesn't mean Type B is to be taken lightly. In 2001, public health officials tracked B/Hong Kong, a rare and serious flu. They were concerned because the notorious strain caused waves of infections in the Northern Hemisphere more than a decade earlier. When it reemerged in 2001, health authorities were alerted to its

---

hemagglutinin

One of the two surface proteins on an influenza virus. Hemagglutinin is important because it is necessary for a flu virus to attach itself to a cell in a host's respiratory system.

neuraminidase

One of the two surface proteins on an influenza virus. Neuraminidase is an enzyme that is essential for flu viruses to spread throughout the respiratory tract.

host

The animal (or human) in which a parasite thrives.

Type B

Pathogen that belongs to the family of orthomyxoviruses. Type B influenza occurs only in humans but can be associated with epidemics. The annual flu vaccine provides protection against one Type B strain.

Influenza 101

presence by a herald wave of infections that moved through parts of Texas and elsewhere in the southwestern United States. A herald wave is defined as a powerful but relatively small number of illnesses. The wave serves as a harbinger of what could occur on a larger scale if infections ultimately involved a greater swath of the population. An aggressive vaccination program helped prevent a major outbreak in 2001.

Aside from its potential to cause outbreaks, Type B influenza has captured the attention of global health officials because it has become resistant in Asia (especially in Japan) to two major antiviral medications. This is a sobering development because it means the drugs have been overused in that part of the world. Should the resistant strains spread beyond Asia (a possibility that is not farfetched), resistance to the same medications can become common elsewhere in the world. If the resistance persists, new medications will have to be developed to treat Type B infections. Even though vaccination is preferred because infection can be prevented, antiviral drugs play an important role, especially in the treatment of patients hospitalized with a flu infection.

Here is a final point to keep in mind about Type B influenza: Just because it is generally less severe than Type A does not mean that it is less prevalent. In some parts of the world, Type B viruses often dominate.

Type C

Pathogen that belongs to the family of orthomyxoviruses. Type C is a much milder form of influenza and manifests as an illness that is very similar to the common cold.

Type C strains can cause outbreaks, but these tend to be dramatically tamer than infections caused by other influenza strains. Type C influenza viruses tend to cause respiratory infections similar to those spurred by viruses that produce the common cold. And because of their tendency to be far tamer than their relatives, public health officials do not provide protection against Type C influenza in the annual vaccine.

A wider range of viruses has been linked to the common cold. More than 200 have been identified. The most common groups of viruses responsible for the illness are **rhinoviruses** and **coronaviruses**, of which there are numerous subtypes. Of these two key groups, rhinoviruses cause from one-third to one-half of all cases of the infection.

The common cold—or catarrh, as it is sometimes called—is far more pervasive than the flu in the number of illnesses it causes. Not only are colds the leading reason adults and children seek a physician's care in the United States, the illness is the primary reason for absences from work and school. Children are far more likely to catch colds than adults, and some estimates indicate that children may catch as many as 9 to 12 colds a year.

Epidemiologists have long thought of schools as incubators of the infection because of the large number of children congregated in them. Scientists also know that the more colds you've had over a lifetime, the less likely you are to catch them as you age. But even though that may seem like good news, the fact remains that no one is ever completely immune to the common cold.

4. How are respiratory infections spread?

Another key similarity between the flu and the common cold is the way in which they are spread. Both respiratory conditions are transmitted through close contact (see **Figure 1**). Droplets of an infected person's secretions, loaded with viruses, become aerosolized—are made airborne—through the explosive forces of coughing and sneezing. These actions can spread the infection to anyone nearby.

If an infected individual doesn't wash after getting these secretions on his or her hands, objects the infected person touches, such as doorknobs or a computer keyboard, can serve as sources of the infection for others who come in contact with them immediately after contamination. Both infections can be spread through an activity as simple as shaking hands.

rhinoviruses
A type of virus that infects the upper respiratory tract and causes the common cold.

coronaviruses
A family of viruses that includes those responsible for the common cold.

Influenza 101

In some instances, an infection can be spread in an activity as simple as holding a conversation with someone at close range. Dr. Marc Siegel in his book, *Bird Flu: Everything You Need to Know About the Next Pandemic,* provides yet another reason why secondhand cigarette smoke is bad for those who inhale

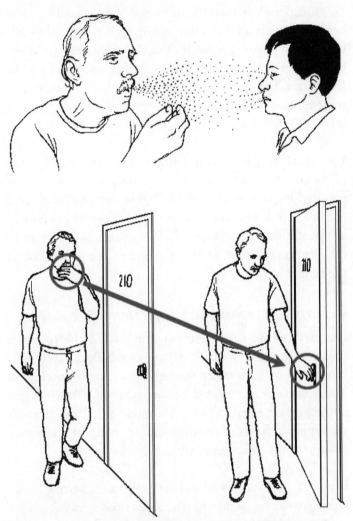

Figure 1   How Does the Flu Spread? The flu spreads in different ways. For example: (a) George has the flu. The flu virus goes into the air when he coughs, sneezes, or talks. If people are nearby, the virus can enter their eyes, nose, and mouth. (b) George coughs into his hand. Then, he touches a doorknob. Now the flu virus is on the doorknob. (continues on next page)

it: He writes that smoke exhaled by an infected person can transmit the flu to anyone nearby.

The flu-spreading actions that have drawn the most study by scientists, as alluded to in Question 1, are coughing and

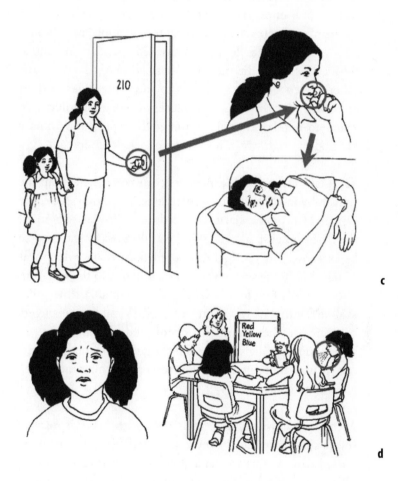

c

d

(c) Later, Geetha touches the doorknob. The virus gets on her hand. The virus gets into her body when she touches her nose. A few days later, Geetha gets sick with the flu. (d) Geetha passes the flu virus to her daughter Sneha. Soon Sneha gets the flu. She can spread the virus to her classmates if she goes to school with the flu.

Courtesy of Government of Alberta © 2008.

sneezing. Both responses are natural in any respiratory disease because they are the overt reactions the body produces to rid itself of infection. When someone is within range of airborne secretions they are likely to inhale viral particles.

As unimaginable as it may seem, endless chains of these simple modes of transmission help spread the flu and colds throughout communities. At a major conference on seasonal and pandemic influenza held in Arlington, Virginia, in February 2007, a leading U.S. flu expert chastised scientists and public health officials at the meeting for shaking hands with each other. He encouraged attendees to adopt the Asian custom of bowing, thereby reducing chances of spreading infections. Hand-to-hand contact, he reminded the experts, is a primary method through which respiratory illnesses are spread.

Yet it isn't just medical experts who are concerned about the transmission of respiratory infections. In March 2007, the captain of a commercial airliner ordered a 16-year-old girl off the flight because her coughing was deemed by the crew to be excessive. The girl had just boarded the plane, which was to take her home to Hawaii after a school trip to New York City and Washington, D.C. The Continental Airlines pilot said he felt that he was acting in the girl's and the passengers' best interest when he ordered her off, and that he didn't want to risk endangering passengers if the girl had something serious. It was discovered that the teen had nothing more than a common cold.

Severe acute respiratory syndrome— SARS—was transported from China to Canada via infected passengers on a plane.

Memories, however, were still fresh of the 2003 spread of severe acute respiratory syndrome—SARS—that was transported from China to Canada via infected passengers on a plane. Additionally, there is a continuing fear that a serious flu strain might be transmitted from one part of the world to another via infected aircraft passengers.

5. What does a flu virus look like? Why do flu viruses usually cause mild to moderate disease, but sometimes cause frightening, large-scale global infections?

Like any virus, those that cause influenza are neither alive nor dead. They survive through an ability to infect their hosts, mutating season-to-season at rates that outpace their hosts' ability to fend them off. Magnified with the aid of an electron microscope, a flu virus looks like a mere fluff of protein stippled with a multitude of tiny spikes. Imagine a miniature mace, the medieval weapon, a metal ball with dozens of spikes—that's basically a flu virus up close and personal. On a flu virus, however, those protrusions are labeled H (hemagglutinin) and N (neuraminidase), the proteins it uses to infect your cells. You may also hear the term surface proteins or surface antigens with respect to flu viruses. The reference in such instances is to H and N, or HA and NA to more precisely indicate the hemagglutinin and neuraminidase of avian influenza viruses (See **Figure 3**).

Below the surface proteins within the viral core lie eight **genes**, which are made up of the genetic material known as ribonucleic acid (RNA). RNA tends to mutate at a faster pace than do genes composed of deoxyribonucleic acid (**DNA**), and that is at least one major reason why flu viruses tend to transform themselves so quickly from one season to the next.

To better understand the kinds of transformations that flu viruses make it is best to get a grasp of the two significant ways in which Nature has endowed these infinitesimal pathogens with an ability to change. Scientists refer to these alterations as **antigenic drift** and **antigenic shift**. Drift refers to the slight changes the virus makes continuously. You might recognize this flux as the tiny changes from one flu season to the next and the reason you are vaccinated every year (See **Figures 2 and 3**).

The antibodies you made against the flu last year after vaccination will not protect you this year because of the drift—the change—in the surface antigens, primarily in H (hemagglutinin).

genes

The basic fundamental units of heredity, each occupying a precise position on a chromosome. Genes are made up of DNA and humans have between 20,000 and 25,000 unique genes.

DNA

Deoxyribonucleic acid is the hereditary chemical that makes up our genes. Humans' genetic information is encoded in DNA.

antigenic drift

Continuous genetic-driven change that causes slight alterations on the surface of flu viruses to outfox the body's immune system, necessitating the need for annual vaccinations.

antigenic shift

A sudden, dramatic genetic change in a dominant circulating Type A influenza virus. The change results in surface antigens that have never before challenged the human immune system.

Influenza 101

Antigenic drift also is the reason that people can catch the flu more than once and are not immune to it after a single bout, as is the case with measles or chicken pox. The tiny alterations flu

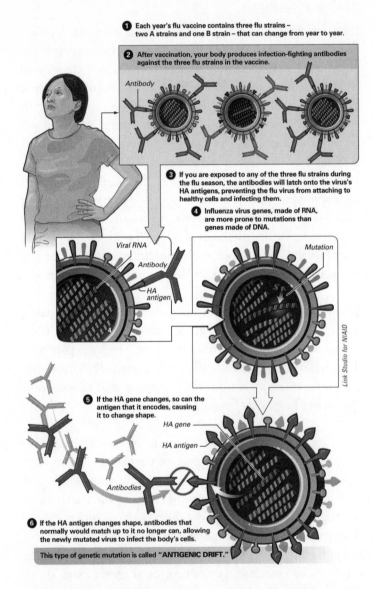

❶ Each year's flu vaccine contains three flu strains – two A strains and one B strain – that can change from year to year.

❷ After vaccination, your body produces infection-fighting antibodies against the three flu strains in the vaccine.

Antibody

❸ If you are exposed to any of the three flu strains during the flu season, the antibodies will latch onto the virus's HA antigens, preventing the flu virus from attaching to healthy cells and infecting them.

❹ Influenza virus genes, made of RNA, are more prone to mutations than genes made of DNA.

Viral RNA

Antibody

Mutation

HA antigen

Link Studio for NIAID

❺ If the HA gene changes, so can the antigen that it encodes, causing it to change shape.

HA gene

HA antigen

Antibodies

❻ If the HA antigen changes shape, antibodies that normally would match up to it no longer can, allowing the newly mutated virus to infect the body's cells.

This type of genetic mutation is called "ANTIGENIC DRIFT."

Figure 2   Antigenic drift. This figure shows how antigenic drift, a mutation of the genes that code for the flu virus's surface antigens, enables a virus to escape or bypass the body's defenses.
National Institute of Allergy and Infectious Diseases (NIAID).

viruses continually make are what allow them to remain infectious. The flu shot you received in previous years does not provide long-lasting protection because the viruses have changed just

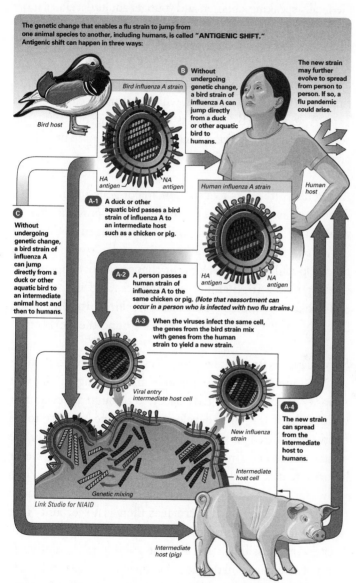

Figure 3 Antigenic shift. This figure shows antigenic shift, the genetic change that enables a flu strain to jump from one animal species to another, including humans.

National Institute of Allergy and Infectious Diseases (NIAID).

Children and younger adults develop a more robust defense against the flu through vaccination than do older adults. But that doesn't mean flu shots are unimportant for people in their 60s or older.

mutation

Any alteration of a gene from its normal sequence of molecular building blocks to a new one.

bird flu

Influenza in wild aquatic birds. Flu viruses in their urine and feces can cause infections with exceptionally high mortality.

enough to be able to penetrate cells in your respiratory tract. Protective antibodies that you produce in response to vaccination generally last only a few months, although there are some notable exceptions, which are explained elsewhere in this book. Generally speaking, children and younger adults develop a more robust defense against the flu through vaccination than do older adults. But that doesn't mean flu shots are unimportant for people in their 60s or older. Getting an annual flu shot helps your immune system mount its most effective attack against flu strains in circulation during the season in which you are vaccinated. Both Type A and Type B flu viruses undergo antigenic drift. And because viruses are constantly changing, it is important to be as prepared as possible for flu season.

Antigenic shift refers to a sudden, major genetic change in a Type A virus. In this kind of **mutation**, the proteins that flu viruses use as tools to infect cells have changed so dramatically that globe-circling waves of illness can sweep through human populations. This kind of change rarely happens, but it can produce frightening consequences and is the reason global health authorities are closely tracking **bird flu**, caused by H5N1 as it moves through flocks around the world.

Surveillance is aimed at keeping an eye on the genetic changes H5N1 undergoes and how people are catching it. The vast majority of human cases have occurred through direct contact with birds. If the virus develops the genetic capacity to be easily transmitted person-to-person, it then is possible for the strain to become a new influenza A subtype that has never before circulated widely among human populations. No one knows for sure if this will happen. Even if the virus does make the genetic change that experts fear, there is no certainty that it will touch off waves of severe human infections. Still, there is a very real possibility that at some point in time, another A strain of influenza will develop the capacity to cause devastating infections that kill millions.

This is an example of antigenic shift: a new and deadly form of influenza A. Antigenic shift, scientists theorize, occurred prior to 1918, triggering the deadliest flu season in the history of humankind.

6. Is influenza a concern worldwide?

Without a doubt, influenza is considered a serious form of respiratory infection around the globe, in nations large and small, and even on remote islands. No region on Earth is immune to influenza. With airlines worldwide moving millions of people daily from one part of the globe to another, it should come as no surprise that contagious illnesses occurring in one part of the world can be easily transported to another in a matter of only a few hours.

But even with information about influenza so readily available from excellent sources, such as the CDC and World Health Organization (**WHO**), which maintain extensive databases on their Web sites, urban legends about global flu transmission patterns still abound. One myth suggests that you can catch the flu only in regions of the world where temperatures dip significantly in winter. The Association for Professionals in Infection Control points out that flu viruses know no boundaries. Because flu viruses are ubiquitous worldwide, the association emphasizes the importance of getting a flu shot before traveling to the Southern Hemisphere between April and September and of being vaccinated regardless of the time of year if you are headed to the tropics.

Scientists at the Fogarty International Center, a division of the National Institutes of Health, have demonstrated how influenza makes its way around the world. The team of virus trackers revealed in a study that influenza tends to travel from low-population regions of the world near the equator to more populated areas.

WHO

World Health Organization; an agency of the United Nations that plays a vital role in a variety of global health concerns.

Influenza 101

The team, led by Dr. Mark Miller, associate director for research at the center, focused on influenza transmission patterns in the Southern Hemisphere and in tropical areas, particularly Brazil. Findings from the research, Miller concludes, can help improve planning for influenza control in sparsely populated regions of the tropics.

Epidemic months in equatorial Brazil occur earlier in the year than they do in the United States and elsewhere in the Northern Hemisphere. But the discovery that influenza tends to move from regions of low population density to crowded urban centers caught scientists off guard. Many had expected the opposite: that the flu would spread first from areas of greater population density. Brazil was chosen not because it is a major source of influenza but because it crosses a broad range of latitudes and encompasses regions that can be considered both tropical and subtropical.

In addition to Miller's research, global health officials are continuously hunting down viral strains circulating worldwide, which means surveillance is conducted in virtually every major region of the globe year-round. Then, in January, based on findings from viral samplings studied in dozens of its global laboratories, the World Health Organization reports the most prominent strains in circulation. The modern ritual of hunting and identifying strains highlights the importance global health authorities give to both the flu and the vaccines that are annually administered to help reduce the amount of influenza circulating in populations. Deactivated snippets from the three most prominent strains (two A and one B) are included in the annual vaccine. Strains included in the vaccines are therefore identical in countries that conduct annual flu vaccinations.

7. Did influenza emerge for the first time in the 20th century?

Influenza is a highly contagious infection that very likely is as old as life itself, having been documented as a seasonal threat throughout much of recorded history. Even when the illness was essentially nameless, societies coped with a season of feverish illness punctuated by sniffles, coughing, and sneezing.

Hippocrates is believed to have recorded the earliest accounts of influenza, highlighting in his writings that the infection is serious and highly contagious. In 412 BC, he described a disease that fueled an **epidemic** so severe it ravaged the Greek army. As epidemiologists would learn in much later years, people in close quarters, such as schools, daycare centers, or military barracks, are much more likely to catch and spread the infection. You may have some idea how rapidly flu outbreaks spread through schools, either because you are a student who became infected along with many of your classmates or you are a parent who has had to nurse more than one child who caught the flu at the same school. No doubt Greek troops were kept huddled closely as they awaited commands, which touched off the epidemic that Hippocrates described.

Hundreds of years later in AD 876, Charlemagne, the King of France, learned the same grim facts about respiratory disease. As he marched from one region of Europe to the next in an attempt to claim the continent for France, his troops were hopelessly crippled by a respiratory infection that experts now believe was influenza. For him, the flu proved as ferocious as the armies that attacked his troops. Medical historians theorize that Charlemagne's soldiers were attempting to claim a major victory for France in the midst of what was very likely a severe flu epidemic. As a war strategy, fighting in the middle of what today is known as flu season couldn't have been more poorly conceived.

Historic references to influenza do not end with Charlemagne and his unfortunate campaign. By the 15th century, the Italians began to discern the seasonal nature of the flu and described its periodicity—the way it arrived unfailingly each winter. As explained in greater detail in Question 8, the

epidemic

Any outbreak of disease in a population that is higher than expected.

Influenza 101

Italians gave the seasonal infection its name. Records also exist describing a late winter illness that spread through the court of England's Elizabeth I, producing symptoms remarkably close to those of influenza.

Between 1830 and 1832, a devastating sweep of influenza spun around the world, killing millions of people. In 1899, an epidemic that spread across Europe awakened an increasingly more modern world to influenza's strength. Known as the Russian flu, medical historians say the infection spread from one region to another with unforeseen force. Like the pandemic that occurred only 19 years later at the close of World War I, the 1899 epidemic caused a stir. Fear permeated populations far and wide as waves of respiratory illness spread from one country to the next. In some countries, historians estimate that up to 50% of the population was stricken by the infection. However, most scientists do not believe the 1899 influenza virus had any link to the one that emerged two decades later and triggered the ferocious pandemic of 1918.

Arriving at the close of World War I, the 1918 outbreak, which is also known as the **Spanish flu**, claimed more lives of military personnel than were killed in the war. Approximately 40 million to 50 million people worldwide died of the flu strain that rapidly circled the globe. This is considered the worst flu season in the history of the world and is defined as the fearsome type of outbreak referred to as a pandemic. Experts believe that more people were killed by the 1918 pandemic than the number who died in Europe's bubonic plague, a rat-borne infectious outbreak that started in 1347 and ran until 1351. The plague left no corner of the continent unscathed, but during the 1918 flu pandemic never had so many people died in so short a time.

At the turn of the 20th century, scientists were much less certain about the illness they called influenza because they were stymied in efforts to identify its cause. Before an actual virus was identified in 1933, theoreticians suggested many different kinds of microorganisms lay at the heart of the disease. **Bacteria**, fungi, and even protozoa were fingered as culprits despite mere circumstantial evidence indicting each.

8. What does the word influenza mean?

Influenza is derived from the Italian word *influentia,* which means to influence. There are two slightly different historical references to the meaning of the word. According to one widely reported explanation, the term refers to an "influence of the stars." As the stars aligned in their positions, arrayed brilliantly in winter's night sky, 15th-century Italian thinkers believed the positions of celestial bodies *influenced* the timing of flu outbreaks.

Other accounts suggest a slightly different meaning. Following an outbreak that sickened thousands in Italy, some references suggest that medieval theorists presumed the illness was caused by an *"influenza di freddo,"* an influence of cold weather. Regardless of which interpretation you find most plausible, the term has survived for many centuries to describe the respiratory illness we refer to as influenza and its shorthand term, the flu.

The infection has gone by other names throughout the course of history and in various parts of the world. *The grippe* is a term that was widely used in the United States in the early years of the 20th century, especially during the 1918 pandemic. Usage of *the grippe* to describe the illness known as influenza has not become passé terminology. In French-speaking Canada and in France, *la grippe* is the preferred term for the flu.

9. What is meant by seasonal flu?

Seasonal flu is the respiratory illness that comes around like clockwork every winter in the Northern Hemisphere and earlier in the year for those who reside south of the equator. Circulating influenza viruses trigger infections, mainly those

bacteria

A vast group of microscopic organisms ubiquitous throughout the world, many of which live on and within humans.

Influenza 101

influenza B

A type of influenza virus capable of triggering epidemics.

that are dubbed H3N2, H1N1, and **influenza B**. H3N2 and H1N1 are both A subtypes. H1N1 is the dramatically milder descendant of the 1918 pandemic strain, the mother of all pandemics, which killed millions of people from as far north as the remote Aleutian villages in the Alaskan permafrost to as far south as the equally remote villages of Africa. Seasonal flu, though serious, does not pose pandemic fears. Severe epidemics, however, can be caused by seasonal flu strains. An epidemic is a severe outbreak in a community—or many communities—at the same time.

In the 2003–2004 flu season, an epidemic was driven by A-Fujian, a subtype of H3N2. The flu season had an unusually early start, as cases were reported in September. The outbreak is most noteworthy for its severity among children. The strain caused a higher-than-usual number of deaths among youngsters, who ranged in age from infancy to teenagers. The earlier start of flu season caught the public health community off guard. Because so many people in the United States were clamoring to be vaccinated, a vaccine shortage quickly emerged.

In the Northern Hemisphere, infections generally occur any time from late November through early March. Respiratory illnesses that occur during summer usually are caused by other pathogens, such as one of the many viruses linked to the common cold. The hallmark of seasonal influenza is its high degree of contagion. The viruses are easily transmitted not only because they can be aerosolized in a cough or sneeze, but also because the pathogens are constantly undergoing change, a factor that ensures contagion (See **Figure 4**).

As a result, people and animals susceptible to illness from influenza infection do not have robust immunity against the mutations that the flu virus produces in very short periods of time. Constant viral mutation drives the need to alter the composition of the annual vaccine. This ensures that each year's vaccine is providing maximum protection against the ever-changing character of influenza viruses. Flu-tracking scientists are constantly taking samples and studying the infections worldwide as a way to keep pace with mutating influenza viruses. Those that are the cause of the largest number of flu cases are usually the ones chosen for the annual vaccine.

Again, influenza infections are passed through close human contact, spreading through chains of coughing and sneezing—in homes, schools, offices, and public places. Seasonal illness can be prevented through vaccination. Additional precautions, such as frequent hand washing and avoidance of hand contact with your nose, mouth, or eyes, especially after shaking hands with anyone, helps limit the possibility of catching the flu.

The influenza vaccine is highly recommended by public health authorities worldwide, especially for people in certain vulnerable age groups. In the United States, the Advisory

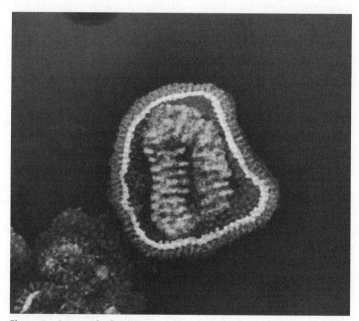

Figure 4   Image of a flu virus.
Courtesy of the Centers for Disease Control and Prevention.

Children and teens on aspirin therapy are advised to get a flu shot as a precaution against Reye's syndrome, a rare condition that can lead to major organ damage and possibly death in kids 15 years old and younger.

Committee on Immunization Practices, a panel of experts that counsels the CDC on vaccine policies, recommends that children between the ages of 6 months and 18 years be vaccinated annually against the flu. The same panel also highly recommends that adults 50 and older receive an annual flu shot. The panel's emphasis is strongest for people 65 and older who are most susceptible to secondary infections that can occur as a result of a flu infection.

Equally high on the committee's list of people in need of annual flu protection are children and adults with medical conditions that impair breathing or compromise immunity. For instance, children and teens on aspirin therapy, usually for arthritis or other inflammatory conditions, are advised to get a flu shot as a precaution against Reye's syndrome, a rare condition that can lead to major organ damage and possibly death in kids 15 years old and younger. The syndrome is marked by brain inflammation and almost always is preceded by a viral illness, such as chickenpox or the flu. Doctors have noted that, even though rare, children on aspirin therapy run a higher than usual risk for Reye's syndrome during flu season. Vaccination, therefore, helps guard against the flu, thwarting the potential for Reye's.

As mentioned earlier, people with respiratory conditions, such as asthma or COPD, should be vaccinated against the flu. But experts also strongly advise that anyone with heart disease, diabetes, HIV infection, or cancer be vaccinated annually against the seasonal infection. A more in-depth examination of who should get vaccinated is in Part 2, "The Flu Shot: Notes on the Only Annual Vaccine."

10. What is avian influenza?

In recent years, global public health officials have been monitoring the spread of an influenza strain circulating in flocks of birds worldwide. The term avian influenza means the same thing as bird flu. There is no difference. The strain that has drawn the spotlight—H5N1—was first identified spreading rapidly among Hong Kong birds in 1997. Gallows humor of the day sometimes referred to the infection as fowl plague to describe the lethal sweep of a strain that had spread among domestic birds. (Sometimes virologists or some newspaper science writers will refer to the bird flu virus as A/H5N1. In so doing, they simply are highlighting that the avian flu virus is an A strain. Again, the *H* stands for hemagglutinin and the *N* for neuraminidase, the two proteins that stipple the virus's surface.)

It is not too difficult to understand how avian influenza—or bird flu, if you prefer that term—became a concern. Influenza viruses are part of the natural gastrointestinal flora of many wild birds. Millions of wild ducks and other waterfowl are native to Asia and harbor various A strains of the virus without becoming ill. Domestic birds, on the other hand, can be mortally sickened by flu strains that their wild cousins live with harmlessly. In 1997, chickens were obvious casualties in a rapidly spreading outbreak in Hong Kong that proved devastating for domestic birds. The avian plague was an initial tip-off to epidemiologists that an unusual—and deadly—flu strain was on the rise.

Yet, H5N1 didn't appear for the first time in 1997, say flu experts, who now believe the strain may have been smoldering among wild birds for more than a century. It is only when domestic birds are sickened and dying in waves that people become alarmed. Italian scientists were the first to report evidence of something very similar as early as 1878. The Italians were also first to invoke the term fowl plague to describe the dramatic waves of death among domestic birds they observed. In 1959, scientists in Scotland became the first to isolate H5N1 following the deaths of chickens affected by a lethal and pervasive infection. By that time, biologists were well aware that wild birds harbored influenza viruses and could transmit them to domestic flocks.

Influenza 101

In the summer of 1997, epidemiologists from the World Health Organization noticed that people in Hong Kong also were being affected. The question was whether humans had contracted the infection directly from birds or whether the strain had acquired the genetic capacity to be easily transmitted from one person to another. If such was the case, scientists knew they were on the cusp of a potentially lethal outbreak. The WHO initially recorded 18 infections of H5N1 in children and adults. Six people died. As far as experts could tell, the infections resulted from direct contact with sick birds.

Within the span of a few months, the infection was diagnosed in a total of 45 children and adults. Mortality was an astonishing 75%. Mounting infections touched off alarms in the global public health community, spurring the CDC to send teams to Hong Kong to investigate. Epidemiologists know that when an avian strain infects domestic birds there are two main forms of infection that can occur: low-level and high-level disease. Technically, these two forms of infection are known as **low-pathogenicity avian influenza** and **high-pathogenicity avian influenza**.

In instances of low-level disease, symptoms may be nothing more than ruffled feathers and a drop in egg production. This form of infection can go unnoticed, even by farmers—for months. But in high-level disease, birds experience multiple organ failure, marked by extreme internal hemorrhaging. Mortality can reach 100% within 48 hours.

In Hong Kong, high-level disease was spreading through domestic flocks. A high-pathogenic form of the virus can remain viable in bird feces for up to 35 days, which means there is ample opportunity for birds to become infected and for humans to come in contact with it on their feet or hands.

H5N1, which never before had infected humans, signaled the potential for a pandemic strain, one that might whip through

---

low-pathogenicity avian influenza

Term used to describe the infectiousness of the avian influenza. Low-pathogenic strains are less lethal than high-pathogenic strains because they do not spread as efficiently or produce high mortality.

high-pathogenicity avian influenza

Term used to describe the infectiousness of the avian influenza. High-pathogenic strains will produce widespread disease in flocks of domestic birds and carry a high death rate.

human populations with unprecedented ferocity and speed. But WHO scientists were quick to caution that this would happen if and only if certain genetic changes occurred within H5N1 that would allow it to be transmitted easily from one person to the next. For such transmission to become possible, avian viral genes might have to intermingle with those of a common human influenza virus, experts said. Sharing of genetic material is common among flu viruses. But if an exchange of genetic material occurred between H5N1 and a common strain that infected humans, the new strain would be imbued with the characteristics of seasonal flu. Seasonal flu is highly contagious and easily transmitted worldwide through close human contact.

Hong Kong government officials ordered a dramatic culling of every kind of bird—millions of birds were killed. Some were thrown into piles on the street and set ablaze. Those efforts seemed to send the strain into retreat. But by 2003, the virus emerged among birds in Southeast Asia, and again, infected a small number of people who had close contact with flocks. Over the next several years, the strain continued to spread rapidly among domestic birds and intermittently infected humans.

Even though human cases were first detected in Southeast Asia, an alarming number of cases were diagnosed in Turkey in 2006. Birds throughout that country were culled in an attempt to prevent viral spread. Turkish citizens had several characteristics in common with those in Vietnam and elsewhere in Southeast Asia where people had become infected with H5N1. Many were rural farmers whose close contact with chickens and other birds suggested the infection was spread from fowl to human.

On a positive note, there is a veterinary vaccine capable of preventing infection in birds, and several more are under study to prevent the infection in humans. Even though the first vaccine for humans against bird flu was not as effective as scientists had hoped, U.S. federal health officials slated it for the **Strategic National Stockpile**, the cache of medications, vaccines, and emergency supplies that are maintained in secret locations throughout the United States. Contents of the strategic stockpile are rolled out in the event of a major catastrophe, such as the attack on the World Trade Center in New York City in 2001 or to aid natural disaster victims, such as those who survived Hurricane Katrina in 2005. Additional vaccines against H5N1 remain under study, including a nasal spray that is composed of live but weakened avian flu viruses.

The veterinary vaccine is not part of the stockpile. It is important, however, because it helps build immunity in birds against H5N1. Studies have demonstrated that immunity against the infection occurs within a week to two weeks after immunization. The vaccine has been administered to chickens because the virus is so lethal and also because of the birds' economic importance. Protection is increased when they receive a booster vaccination within 8 to 10 weeks of the initial inoculation. As you might imagine, this form of protection is very expensive but cannot prevent the global spread of the virus. Wild birds, especially ducks, are carriers of the infection and their range along well-traveled global "flyways" takes them on a migration path that is very broad.

Poultry farmers go to great lengths to protect domestic birds by vaccinating them against H5N1, but wild, migrating ducks can swoop down to steal food and mingle with domestic flocks before resuming their journey. Ducks are well known for leaving behind tokens of their visit—virus-laden feces that can infect chickens.

Even though farmers, particularly in China and Southeast Asia, are using the vaccine to immunize chickens, problems still abound with this form of protection. The vaccination does not always work and birds have become infected with

---

Strategic National Stockpile

The stockpile is organized and controlled by the Center is for Disease Control and Prevention and is designed as a national repository of antibiotics, vaccines, medications, life-support equipment, and medical and surgical supplies.

Wild birds, especially ducks, are carriers of the infection and their range along well-traveled global "flyways" takes them on a migration path that is very broad.

H5N1 despite preventive efforts. Currently, the avian vaccine is injected, but studies are under way to develop a spray, which could distribute the vaccine faster and to more birds in a single application. Unfortunately, the technology to administer vaccinations in this way has yet to be developed and approved, and therefore probably will not be available in the near future.

11. Is H5N1 the only "bird flu" strain under scientific investigation?

Because birds are the natural reservoir of influenza viruses, many strains have captured scientific attention—all of them because they have proved to be lethal in domestic birds. Among the other strains under close scrutiny are H7N7, another "bird flu," or avian strain. The National Influenza Center in the Netherlands has since 2003 reported several dozen human infections triggered by H7N7. Most of the cases have occurred among poultry workers who had close contact with birds.

Even though farmers are using the vaccine to immunize chickens, problems still abound with this form of protection. The vaccination does not always work and birds have become infected with H5N1 despite preventive efforts.

The virus does not appear to be as lethal in humans as H5N1. However, a 57-year-old veterinarian who had visited one of the poultry farms where chickens were severely stricken died of **acute respiratory distress syndrome (ARDS)**. Dutch health authorities also report that poultry workers have transmitted this form of bird flu to family members. Human-to-human cases have been limited, but scientists are very concerned about H7N7. Like H5N1, H7N7 is subject to mutations that might produce a deadly strain. The virus is under intense study in laboratories throughout Europe, Canada, and the United States. In addition to the deaths of chickens in the Netherlands, H7N7 also has caused poultry deaths in Belgium and Germany. Vaccines are under study.

acute respiratory distress syndrome (ARDS)

Can occur as a result of infections, injuries, or other conditions that cause the lung's capillaries to leak more fluid than normal into the alveoli (the air sacs of the lungs).

Another bird flu virus that has captured a spotlight is H9N2, a pathogen that apparently is endemic to ducks. It has spread to other forms of poultry in Asia. Between 1999 and 2003,

Influenza 101

29

the strain caused illnesses in three children who live in Hong Kong. Human infections did not appear again until 2007 when a 9-month-old baby developed the flu caused by this unusual strain. The National Institutes of Health in the United States supports research on a vaccine against H9N2 by the Chiron Corporation, of Emeryville, California.

12. How are flu viruses transmitted among birds and from birds to humans?

Droppings from infected birds, as mentioned in Question 10, are loaded with live flu viruses. Domestic birds are often susceptible to inhaling viruses contained in feces. People who handle the birds and who get fecal matter on their hands are also highly susceptible to infection. A majority of human cases involving H5N1, H7N7, and H9N2 involve close contact with infected domestic birds and their feces or the feces of migrating wild birds that are left in a domestic flock's pen.

A majority of human cases involving H5N1, H7N7, and H9N2 involve close contact with infected domestic birds and their feces or the feces of migrating wild birds that are left in a domestic flock's pen.

13. What is pandemic influenza?

Pandemic influenza is the flu in its most dreaded form, the kind of severe infection with rapid spread and high mortality driven by a Type A strain that has never before entered the human population. Public health experts who monitor the progression of avian influenza as it spreads among birds fear the virus will mutate into a form that can be transmitted to humans with a potential to trigger a pandemic. They closely study human cases of bird flu to determine how the disease is transmitted.

Pandemic is the word invariably used to describe the 1918 flu outbreak or the two later 20th-century globe-circling outbreaks, the 1957 Asian flu and the Hong Kong flu of 1968. Dr. Michael Osterholm, an epidemiologist and influenza expert at the University of Minnesota, estimates that 10 highly virulent outbreaks, driven by a Type A strain, have swept around the world over the past 300 years. In an article in the *New England*

Journal of Medicine in May 2005, Osterholm noted that many flu experts believe the 1918 flu to be an anomaly, standing out as the most severe spate of lethal flu infections in the history of the world. But a flu pandemic that struck between 1830 and 1832 was similarly devastating, according to Osterholm. The difference between the 19th-century pandemic and the one that occurred in 1918 was population size. Global population was significantly smaller in the 1830s, which made the flu's impact seem less devastating. Today with a global population of 6.5 billion, more than three times the number of people alive in 1918, even a relatively mild pandemic could kill tens of millions of people if a deadly strain were to emerge.

Many epidemiologists believe the world is long overdue for another large-scale influenza pandemic. Virologists are certain that pandemic strains circle the globe periodically. What they have been unable to predict is the *periodicity*, the timing from one pandemic to another, if such timing can be forecast at all. Walter Dowdle of the Task Force for Child Survival and Development wrote in a 2006 issue of the journal *Emerging Infectious Diseases* that epidemiologists have long tried to determine whether pandemics can be predicted. Having such knowledge in hand would allow governments sufficient time to prepare for a potentially killer outbreak. But Dowdle writes: "The exact conditions that lead to the emergence of a pandemic strain are still unknown."

For many years, some scientists thought that pandemics occurred in periods every 10 to 11 years. The 1968 Hong Kong Flu came exactly 11 years after the 1957 Asian flu. As a result, there was little surprise in 1976 when then-President Gerald Ford announced on March 24, 1976, that preparedness was vital for a strain that seemed to be gathering strength. Government health experts dubbed the strain Swine flu. Said Ford: "No one knows exactly how serious this threat could be. Nevertheless, we cannot afford to take a chance with the nation's health." The president urged public health experts to mount an aggressive nationwide vaccination campaign. Television, newspapers, and magazines revived images of the 1918 pandemic and warned of a threat so dire that one would be foolish to avoid vaccination against the superstrain of flu that was certain to make its way around the globe (See **Figure 5**).

But an outbreak of the proportions for which government officials braced never came to be. Indeed, the vaccine itself caused problems in at least 50 immunized people, all of whom developed **Guillain-Barre syndrome**, a condition in which the immune system attacks parts of the nervous system. Many who suffer from the syndrome experience weakness and a pins-and-needles sensation in their legs. In time, the weakness can spread and, for some people, affected muscles become useless. In such instances, the disorder becomes life threatening. At least six people vaccinated against Swine flu died.

Guillain-Barre syndrome

A rare disorder involving an attack on the nervous system by turncoat constituents of the immune system.

The failure of Swine flu to materialize into a global outbreak did not disrupt attempts to predict pandemics. Scientists now have turned to sophisticated computer modeling applications in an effort to better understand the cycles in which pandemic strains have entered human populations. The studies have at least assured researchers of one undeniable fact: Flu pandemics have occurred in the past and are certain to occur in the future.

14. So far, there has been no mention of stomach flu or the 24-hour "flu bug." Are these infections genuine influenza?

Just about everyone at some point has either said—or heard someone else say—"I've got stomach flu," or "I've got a 24-hour flu bug." Both terms are so widely used that virtually everyone probably thinks there are reams of medical data on how the influenza virus causes gastrointestinal problems.

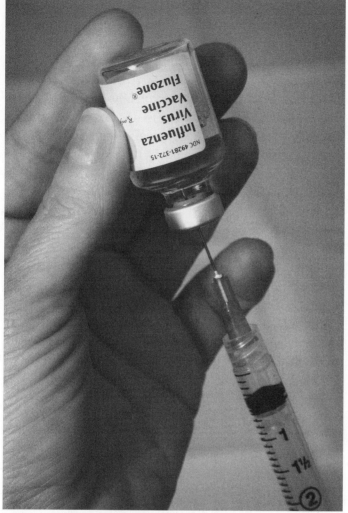

Figure 5   The flu vaccine being extracted from a 5-mL vial.
Courtesy of the Centers for Disease Control and Prevention.

As it turns out, neither the stomach flu nor the so-called 24-hour flu bug have anything to do with influenza. In fact, both terms refer to a single illness, which doctors would most likely diagnose as gastroenteritis. It is typified by severe stomach and intestinal distress caused primarily by a bacterial infection. These illnesses almost always can be traced to tainted food or contaminated water. Food- and waterborne illnesses are a significant cause of sickness—and death—in the United States. But even if you think that you may be affected by stomach flu, influenza virus is not the cause.

Again, influenza is a respiratory condition caused by any of the viral strains circulating in a given season. Fever, malaise, and chills are some of the symptoms experienced during a bout with the flu, and interestingly, they are the same symptoms that can occur with gastroenteritis. But that is where the similarities end. Anyone affected with gastroenteritis also experiences vomiting and diarrhea. Diarrhea can become so severe in some cases that the person becomes dehydrated and must be hospitalized. Certain foodborne infectious agents are noteworthy because some bacteria produce a toxin, as is the case with *Escherichia coli* O157:H7. In extreme cases, the bacterial toxin can lead to red blood cell damage and kidney failure. *E. coli*, as the pathogen is more commonly known, has captured a spotlight in recent years because of its presence in contaminated beef, spinach and lettuce.

Gastroenteritis, however, can be triggered by any one of several pathogenic bacteria. Among them are *Salmonella*, which can taint eggs or chicken; *Campylobacter*, another bacterial contaminant of chicken; *Shigella*, a fecal bacterium transmitted when an infected food handler has not washed his or her hands; and, of course, *E. coli* O157:H7, a bovine fecal bacterium.

Despite the complete lack of a relationship between the influenza virus and the bacteria that cause gastroenteritis, public health experts doubt the terms "stomach flu" and "24-hour flu bug" will disappear anytime soon.

PART TWO

The Flu Shot: Notes on the Only Annual Vaccine

What should I know about the annual flu vaccine?

How are the annual flu shots made?

I've heard about a universal flu vaccine.
What is it and how does it work?

More . . .

15. What is a vaccine?

Generally speaking, a vaccine is a preparation composed of the entire organism or fragments of the infectious agent. The organism can be **inactivated** (killed) or **attenuated** (live, but weakened). Both types, which are discussed in greater detail elsewhere in this section, are administered in each year's flu vaccination campaign. The purpose of a vaccine is to induce immunity against the disease that the organism causes, and thus protect you from getting sick. Vaccination does not intervene in a disease already in progress. Instead, a vaccine prompts your immune system to produce its own forces to prevent infection from occurring in the first place. One of the most important points to understand about vaccines is that they do not function like medications. Immunization against the flu is the only form of vaccination that is offered on an annual basis. As mentioned earlier, flu viruses mutate at an extraordinarily high rate of speed and because of that it is important to produce a new vaccine to account for changes flu viruses make from one season to the next.

inactivated

An infective agent that has lost its disease-producing capacity.

attenuated

A vaccine made up of bacteria or viruses of the infection that is to be prevented through vaccination.

16. Against which flu viruses do seasonal vaccines provide protection?

Seasonal flu vaccines are produced every year to provide protection against circulating strains. Flu viruses are tricky. If people were able to mount permanent immunity after a single bout with the infection, no one would ever have to worry about catching the flu again—or being vaccinated. But because of the constant state of change of flu viruses no one can ever be permanently immune.

Virus hunters from WHO, CDC, and other global health agencies track the prevalence of key influenza subtypes. H3N2, H1N1, and influenza B are always on their radar. Generally, any one of the numerous variations of these viruses is included in the trivalent flu vaccine that is administered annually. A trivalent vaccine is made up of three components.

The subtypes that are most prevalent and causing the most infections are usually the ones selected to be included in the annual vaccine. Question 24 addresses additional details about seasonal flu viruses and vaccines.

17. Is there any other important information on how vaccines work?

When a virus causes an infection, it introduces its proteins, or **antigens**, into your cells. Vaccination introduces an infinitesimal amount of viral antigens into your body. Keep in mind that the amount of antigens introduced into the body is far too small to cause the disease. The important aspect to grasp is that when your immune system recognizes the presence of these antigens, it immediately memorizes these invaders and counteracts them by producing **antibodies**. These tiny proteins are generated by white blood cells and are capable of neutralizing antigens.

Vaccination is important because if you encounter flu viruses at any time during flu season, your immune system can respond by producing a torrent of antibodies that are already primed against the specific strains in circulation. Your immune system is able to do this because it stores information about the antigens when you are vaccinated. Highly specific antibodies are therefore capable of binding to the antigens (which are on the viral surface) and destroying the entire virus. This incredible activity is part of the intricate functions of the human immune system and basically describes what is meant by the term **immune response**.

Antibodies do not only provide protection against the flu. They are mounted when the immune system recognizes *any* viruses, bacteria, or toxins that invade the body. What turns out to be one of the true marvels of biology is the high degree of specificity that antibodies have. Antibodies marshaled against influenza fight only flu viruses; antibodies that marshal against polio fight only that virus. Antibodies are so specialized that each

antigens

Any foreign substance that, when introduced into the body, stimulates an immune response, causing the body to release antibodies.

antibodies

A Y-shaped protein that is made by the body's immune system in response to non-invasive foreign substances, such as bacteria, viruses, protozoa, fungi, toxins, and even transplanted organs.

immune response

The immune system's reaction to infection, toxins, or transplanted organs.

responds only to specific foreign particles that find their way into your system. This specificity is why the antibodies coaxed by the flu vaccine of one year provide no protection next flu season because the flu virus tweaks its own surface proteins—its antigens—during its continual state of mutation. You, therefore, must prime your immune system through vaccination each year to be fully immunized against flu strains in circulation.

With all of this in mind, it should come as no surprise that antigens are the key components of a vaccine. When your immune system encounters the foreign antigens contained in the vaccine it begins marshaling forces against them. Vaccines are administered in tiny doses because nothing greater is needed to prompt your body to fight infectious invaders. One theory behind vaccination is simple: You won't be caught off guard. Of course there are notable exceptions, which are discussed elsewhere in this book. But the take-home message is easy to understand: Should you encounter an infection for which you have already been administered a vaccine you should remain disease-free because your body has already mounted a hardy defense against the condition, allowing you to resist it.

Influenza probably will not be eradicated—certainly not anytime soon—because it is caused by several strains of the influenza virus that all mutate at a relatively high rate.

Vaccines exist for a wide variety of infectious microbes that once plagued humans and domestic animals. Indeed, they've played key roles in the control and elimination of many devastating infections. For example, smallpox was completely eradicated from human populations as a result of an aggressive global vaccination campaign that began in the late 1960s. By 1977, the last case was diagnosed, and in 1980 the World Health Organization officially declared smallpox eradicated. Unfortunately, there are no vaccines for a large number of highly infectious diseases, despite years of research and attempts to make such immunizations reality. Influenza probably will not be eradicated—certainly not anytime soon—because it is caused by several strains of the influenza virus that all mutate at a relatively high rate. Vaccination, however, can control influenza in populations.

18. What should I know about the annual flu vaccine?

The annual flu vaccine can be taken in one of two ways, either as a shot or as a nasal spray. With either form of vaccination, it takes about 2 weeks for your body to mount a sufficient supply of infection-fighting antibodies to prevent infection.

Most people are familiar with the shot in the upper arm. In this case, the vaccine is made up of the inactivated virus strains that are causing influenza during a given flu season. A flu shot contains protection against two Type A strains of flu and one Type B virus. Flu shots can be given to most people who want to be protected from catching the flu.

The CDC has developed a list of "priority groups" who benefit most from a flu shot and who should be among those vaccinated each year. The CDC provides the following information on who should be vaccinated annually:

1. Children 6 months to 18 years old
2. Pregnant women
3. Anyone 50 years old or older
4. Anyone with a chronic medical condition (asthma, COPD, cystic fibrosis, diabetes, HIV infection, or anyone who is receiving chemotherapy for cancer)
5. Residents of nursing homes and other long-term care facilities
6. Household contacts of people at elevated risk of flu complications
7. Household contacts and out-of-home caregivers of children less than 6 months old (these babies are too young to be vaccinated)
8. Healthcare workers

There is also a list of who should *not* receive the shot or the inhaled vaccine: Anyone who has a history of Guillain-Barre syndrome should not be vaccinated. The CDC also suggests that anyone who has a severe allergic reaction to eggs should not get a flu shot because (as is discussed in greater detail in Question 21) doses of the annual flu shot are produced in eggs.

Like the flu shot, the inhaled version is administered in an extremely tiny dose and is made up of the same major strains in circulation for the season. Yet, unlike the flu shot, the nasal spray is composed of live but extraordinarily weakened Type A and Type B strains.

Technically, the nasal spray, sold under the brand name Flu-Mist, is known as an LAIV, which stands for live attenuated influenza vaccine. It was approved by the Food and Drug Administration in 2003 and is produced by MedImmune, Inc., a biotechnology company in Gaithersburg, Maryland. When sprayed into the nose, the vaccine, like its injected counterpart, stimulates the immune system to produce antibodies. Because the nasal vaccine is made up of live but weakened viruses, it is somewhat more complex than the flu shot.

The nasal spray also is defined as a cold-adapted and temperature-sensitive vaccine. This means the weakened viruses in the vaccine can be in the nasal passages and throat long enough for the body to recognize the antigens and produce protective antibodies. The vaccine does not cause the flu for two reasons: the viruses in the vaccine are weakened and the temperature in the respiratory tract is too high for these already altered viruses to be infectious.

Research on weakened, cold-adapted influenza viruses date back to the 1960s when Dr. Hunein F. Maassab of the University of Michigan laid the scientific groundwork for the nasal spray that ultimately would become known as FluMist. Dr. Maassab found that when extremely weakened, the flu virus does not mutate and does not cause the flu. FluMist is recommended only for healthy people between the ages of 5 and 49 years. Additional research could change the eligible age range, expanding the number of people who qualify for this form of vaccination.

Even though clinical studies have shown FluMist does not cause the flu, can close contact with a vaccinated person result in the infection? Generally, that answer is no. But the CDC recommends that anyone who is caring for someone with a severely impaired immune system not be vaccinated with the nasal spray. The advice is a precautionary measure because of the extreme vulnerability of those whose immune systems are not intact.

A final note: The nasal spray, unlike the flu shot, does not contain the preservative thimerosal, which might make it seem a more attractive choice for those who are concerned about the use of the additive in vaccines.

19. How important is the influenza vaccine?

Most who are vaccinated annually against influenza probably focus on one major benefit: Chances are very much in their favor that they won't catch the flu. Public health authorities, on the other hand, take a far broader view. As more people take this preventive measure during any given flu season, the overall burden of influenza declines in the population. In the event of a serious outbreak, its severity is lessened because fewer people can catch and pass along the infection.

Public health policies in the United States and elsewhere in the world have been shaped around the vaccine because it has helped prevent countless cases of the flu in people of all ages. Most adults in Western countries are probably familiar with the annual public health announcements about the benefits of being vaccinated. Epidemiologists have been convinced of the vaccine's overall efficacy as a vital public health tool, based on 70 years of clinical and observational studies.

As with any medical intervention, influenza vaccination is not 100% effective. Studies suggest the vaccine is anywhere from

70% to 90% effective in healthy adults under the age of 65. Among seniors, whose immunity is not as robust as that of younger adults, the vaccine may not always prevent infection. Physicians, nevertheless, are certain that vaccination will at the very least reduce the severity of illness for those 65 and older in the event infection does occur.

One obstacle to lowering the flu's prevalence each season has been convincing enough people of all ages to take part in each year's vaccination campaign. In the United States, anywhere from 80 million to 110 million vaccine doses are produced annually to immunize people nationwide. Despite a concerted push by the federal government to encourage flu vaccination, a significant portion of each season's vaccines is trashed. The practice has come under fire because some public health experts contend that even with minute genetic changes in flu viruses, the millions of unused doses may still be of benefit, particularly for poorer nations that cannot afford to produce their own vaccines. Moreover, the doses themselves are still viable and perfectly safe to be administered. Some scientists estimate that the vaccines remain stable for at least 3 to 4 years. Yet even in the face of such arguments, a ritual as common as the annual autumn vaccination campaign itself has been the destruction of millions of unused doses in early summer.

For example, at midnight June 30, 2007, a date set by the Food and Drug Administration, more than 10 million doses were destroyed. The old doses had to be disposed of before a new round of vaccines could be guaranteed. In addition to arguments that favor donating the vaccines to poorer nations, some health policy analysts suggest allowing doctors to keep vaccines on hand after June in the event travelers to the Southern Hemisphere may want to be vaccinated between July and September. New vaccines—those for the next season—usually are not available until late summer or sometimes even early fall.

Wasted doses have been a primary reason many pharmaceutical companies have abandoned or chosen not to join the flu vaccine production business. The paucity of manufacturers has been of major concern to the National Institutes of Health and the Centers for Disease Control and Prevention. Both agencies have tried to encourage more companies to produce flu vaccines in the event of a severe outbreak or, worse still, a pandemic. In either instance, vaccine production would have to be quickly ramped up to meet the increased demand.

20. Is the flu shot the world's first vaccine?

Influenza vaccination has a long and storied past, beginning with U.S. military efforts aimed at developing an effective form of immunization shortly before World War II. The flu shot, however, is not the world's first vaccine. That distinction belongs to the smallpox vaccine, which was developed somewhat serendipitously in 1796 by Edward Jenner (although many historical accounts suggest the ancient Chinese had developed the practice of smallpox vaccination hundreds of years prior to Jenner's work). Jenner invented the word *vaccination*, which is derived from the Latin word *vacca* for cow. He noticed that milkmaids, who had been exposed to cowpox, an infection specific to cows, never developed smallpox, the leading cause of human death in the 18th century. Viruses caused both cowpox and smallpox, but neither Jenner nor other doctors of his day knew that viruses existed—or triggered either condition.

Jenner knew through his simple observations that cowpox caused a decidedly simpler disease in cows and that because the milkmaids were in contact with the cows' crusted sores they miraculously remained free of smallpox infection. Jenner also was aware that once exposed to cowpox, milkmaids were immune to smallpox for life. He decided to use the crusted matter from the cows as a treatment to prevent smallpox. Jenner's keen scientific insight paved the way for the use of vaccines as major public health tools. Vaccination campaigns based on his inoculation process were under way in Britain as well as the United States by the early 19th century.

Development of the flu vaccine began in earnest in 1941, a day before the United States entered World War II. Military officials established the Commission on Influenza and quickly expanded their effort into a panel known as the Armed Forces Epidemiological Board, which exists to this day. At the time, the hope was to develop a protective vaccine and avoid the devastating flu infections that killed thousands of U.S. troops at the close of World War I.

By the start of World War II, scientists knew without question that the killer influenza, which swept through barracks and ships during World War I, was caused by a virus. Having this knowledge available made it possible for them to think about quickly developing a vaccine. Because of the urgency to thwart what some speculated might be a repeat of the 1918 disaster, the combined talents of military and nonmilitary scientists enabled the first successful field trials of a vaccine by 1943. The surprise for many in the military was that a pandemic did not emerge.

21. How are the annual flu shots made?

Technology involved in manufacturing the annual flu shot dates back to the mid-1940s when doses were first mass-produced for the public. The process is long, laborious, and requires a mind-boggling supply of fertilized hen's eggs, more than 100 million are needed to meet the U.S. government's vaccine dose requirements. In recent years, health officials from the CDC and the National Institute of Allergy and Infectious Diseases (a division of the National Institutes of Health) have complained about the time-consuming process and have supported research investigating more efficient methods of production. As it stands now, it takes about 6 months for seasonal flu vaccines to be manufactured. This doesn't include the time it takes for viral surveillance conducted by a global network of laboratories, which tracks and identifies the most infectious strains in circulation.

The process begins with the collection of viral samples from people sick with the flu in various parts of the world. A surveillance network consisting of 180 laboratories in 83 countries, including the CDC in the United States, is involved in the hunt for the year's most infectious strains. The World Health Organization, which is based in Geneva, coordinates the viral surveillance effort. In the United States, the CDC receives viral isolates from state health department laboratories throughout the country as well as from around the world. CDC scientists then determine which among the pathogens they've received are the most likely candidates to cause influenza in the upcoming flu season. That information is shared with the Food And Drug Administration (FDA) and the WHO. Between January and March, the FDA, CDC, and WHO decide which strains will be included in the vaccine for the upcoming flu season.

As the viral selection process is under way, the four licensed vaccine manufacturers in the United States are preparing for production, and that means buying enough eggs—millions of them—to produce the doses of influenza vaccine. This process strongly relies on the availability of healthy hens to lay the eggs. (Manufacturers do not prepare the viral material that is used to make the vaccines. FDA scientists perform that task.)

Once manufacturers receive the viral material, they begin a production process that has undergone few basic changes since the World War II era. Eleven days after each egg is fertilized it is injected through the shell with the viral preparation. The mixture goes into the fluid surrounding the chick embryo. The embryos become infected, which allows the virus to multiply. After incubating for several days, the fluid is extracted. The viral material is inactivated and purified. Federal health officials estimate that between one and two eggs are required to produce a single dose of flu vaccine. As effective as this process has been for decades in nonemergencies, experts say far less time and up to 10 times the current output would be needed if a deadly flu strain were to emerge. In addition to the amount of time it takes to produce the vaccine, many top public health officials worry that countless lives could be lost in a pandemic if manufacturers were forced to depend on an antiquated egg-based method of production.

22. Are there other ways to make flu shots?

High-tech production methods have been used for years to produce other types of vaccines, which is why public health officials know that egg-based technology does not have to be the sole production method for flu shots. Vaccines can be produced through **cell culture** and genetic technology. Cell culture production involves manufacturing flu vaccines in gigantic vats—fermenters—something akin to what is used to brew beer. This technique relies on cells as the medium in which the vaccines are produced.

cell culture

Term used in reference to the cultivation and maintenance of cells in laboratory.

Protein Sciences, a vaccine manufacturing company in Meriden, Connecticut, was the first to sponsor large-scale clinical studies of a flu vaccine produced in caterpillar cells. The company's small initial batch of vaccines (for the 2008–2009 flu season) marks the first major contribution to public health by the lowly army worm, a leaf-eating caterpillar. Executives at Protein Sciences expect a much larger number of vaccines to be produced in subsequent years. The process does not require the use of live flu viruses as with eggs, and neither does it involve the use of thimerosal, a vaccine preservative that has raised the ire of anti-vaccine organizations.

Vaccines that rely on **genetic technology** involve injecting an infinitesimal snippet of viral genetic material into people. This is done instead of using whole inactivated viruses as with conventional flu shots, or weakened live viruses, as is the case with FluMist. Clinical trials have not yet definitively shown that genetic technology will result in a commercial product any time soon. Studies still could take many years. However, scientists are actively moving ahead with research aimed at providing influenza vaccines produced through methods that do not focus on eggs.

Dr. John Treanor, a vaccine expert at the University of Rochester in upstate New York, said eggs can prove very cumbersome to work with. When millions of fertilized eggs are involved in vaccine production, a host of agricultural issues come to the fore, not to mention concerns involving the handling of flu viruses. Flu viruses, according to Treanor, can be temperamental and it is not always a simple task to get viruses to grow as needed in eggs.

Treanor led a successful study of the vaccine called FluBlOk, the vaccine produced in caterpillar cells. Reporting in the *Journal of the American Medical Association* (April 2007), Treanor and colleagues demonstrated that vaccines, developed through newer and more efficient technology, can be very effective. The scientists tested the vaccine in 460 adult volunteers between the ages of 18 and 49 who received one of three types of flu shots: a high or low dose produced through the insect cells or a placebo that provided no protection. None of the volunteers who received the highest dose became ill with the flu; two who were injected with a low dose came down with it; and seven who received the placebo caught the flu.

The cell line from which the culture is drawn has the potential to reproduce itself indefinitely. In the event of a severe outbreak, vaccine manufacturers can begin production shortly after an infectious strain is fully identified. There would be nothing to interfere with production, such as waiting for hens to lay a sufficient supply of eggs.

Eliminating egg-based production is important for a variety of reasons. People who are allergic to egg proteins can be vaccinated against influenza. Cell culture production is also less time consuming. Treanor estimates that cell culture technology could shave 2 months off the vaccine manufacturing process. In the event of a public health emergency, vaccine production could be ramped up much more quickly.

With FluBlOk, caterpillars did not have to be killed for scientists to retrieve their cells. To start the culture, only a smattering of insect cells was required. Then, under laboratory-controlled conditions, a few were coaxed to produce millions—far more cells than could be retrieved through sacrificing insects. Other types of cell cultures are also being considered, including those based on human stem cells.

23. Does the flu vaccine cause influenza?

Among the unfortunate myths long in circulation about flu vaccination, none are as prevalent as the belief that flu shots cause the flu. As with any form of vaccination, a flu shot can cause a degree of irritation in some sensitive people. Your arm may ache in the spot where the shot was administered; you may feel particularly tired for a day or so after vaccination; you may even run a very mild fever. These are responses your body is making to the vaccine, not signs that you are coming down with the flu. There is, however, the possibility of a coincidental situation that might occur if you choose to be vaccinated during the height of flu season when viruses are in circulation. It is possible to catch the flu shortly before or after you've been vaccinated. A natural instinct is to blame the vaccine. But a flu shot cannot cause the infection, because as mentioned earlier, it is made of inactivated viral particles, not live, highly active ones. Remember, it takes two weeks to mount a defense after vaccination.

Even in the case of FluMist, there is no convincing evidence that weakened influenza viruses cause infection. MedImmune, manufacturer of the FluMist nasal spray vaccine, underscored that in clinical trials of its product there were no cases of influenza triggered by the immunization. That is one reason why medical scientists embarked on a bold experiment in 2006, administering a "live but weakened" vaccine spray against bird flu to healthy volunteers. Bird flu, caused by the H5N1 strain, can be quickly lethal. But when the virus is severely crippled, a more robust form of immunity against the infection can be achieved. To arrive at this end, a weakened form of the virus must be the immunizing component in the vaccine.

24. Does the seasonal flu vaccine always perfectly match the most infectious strains in circulation?

As diligently as virus hunters worldwide work to track down infectious strains and gather information on those causing influenza, the vaccine is not always a perfect match with strains circulating during any given flu season. Each year, as mentioned in Question 16, the flu vaccine (both the shot and nasal spray) contain protection against H3N2, H1N1, and influenza B. Subtypes of these viruses exist all over the world, each with their own nuances and all of them—no matter where they are—in a constant state of flux.

Just for illustrative purposes, let's say virus trackers identify A-California as the major H3N2 subtype causing extensive cases of seasonal influenza; therefore, it is the one chosen for the vaccine. But what if A-Fujian turns out to be the form of H3N2 actually causing serious infections during the season. Does that mean the vaccine is now worthless?

Similar mismatches have occurred in actual flu seasons, but infectious disease specialists say there is no need for alarm. Even when the vaccine does not precisely match the dominant strain of H3N2, studies have demonstrated that people who are vaccinated tend to fare better than those who were not immunized. Annual drifts (mutations) produce viruses that are first cousins of each other, which means the vaccine will help your body mount a defense, although probably not as

Annual drifts (mutations) produce viruses that are first cousins of each other, which means the vaccine will help your body mount a defense.

robust a defense as it would if the match between vaccine and circulating viruses was perfect. However, experts suggest that among people between the ages of 5 and 49 who receive the nasal spray vaccine, there is a strong likelihood of protection in seasons involving a mismatch.

In instances when the infection occurs among those who have received a shot, the bout is likely to be much milder. Bear in mind that seasonal strains differ only slightly from one year to the next. Public health authorities recommend changing the vaccine each year to provide those who are vaccinated with optimum protection. The vaccines are guarding against minor changes resulting from antigenic drift, which occurs in influenza viruses season to season.

25. Would the seasonal vaccine protect against a pandemic flu strain?

The vaccination you receive each year for the flu is against those strains passed commonly among people: H3N2, H1N1, and influenza B. A pandemic strain is one that has never before occurred in the human population; therefore, none of the seasonal vaccine's components have any potency against a new and potentially lethal virus.

Surveillance by global health authorities is riveted on suspect strains that have the potential to enter the human population. Again, that is why WHO, CDC, and European public health agencies are closely monitoring a number of bird flu viruses. In the event that one does cause significant cases of human influenza, work can begin immediately on developing a vaccine specific to that strain.

26. I've heard about a universal flu vaccine. What is it and how does it work?

Vaccinating people against the flu would be much simpler if only one shot was needed, with perhaps a booster dose every few years. Even better would be manufacturing this new kind of flu shot in a cell culture or by way of some other advanced technique, avoiding the need for millions of chicken eggs. Remarkably, scientists are on the trail of such a goal. Researchers at Acambis, a major vaccine manufacturer that is headquartered in Great Britain with U.S. offices in Cambridge, Massachusetts, has been working on a type of vaccination that would end the autumn ritual of getting your annual flu shot.

The flu vaccination under development is known as a **universal vaccine**. It is being designed as a one-time shot with a periodic booster. Current influenza vaccines are changed from year to year because viruses in the wild are constantly altering the character of their surface proteins. As mentioned earlier, the proteins (hemagglutinin and neuraminidase, H and N) are in constant flux. Instead of these two well-known proteins, the universal vaccine could be based on a flu viral protein called **M2-e**, a less widely known component of Type A and B influenza viruses.

M2-e has attracted intense scientific attention because it is more "highly conserved" than the other two proteins. The term highly conserved means that M2-e remains relatively stable and does not change as formidably as H and N do. Some scientists speculate that because M2-e is so stable, a vaccine that is based on it would probably work well enough to prevent seasonal *and* pandemic influenza. But even in the face of such alluring theories the universal flu vaccine is still years away.

M2-e has been an object of intense research in the United States as well as in the European Union where Belgian, Dutch,

universal vaccine
A flu vaccine that can be administered against any seasonal strain as well as serve as a preventive against any emergent pandemic strain.

M2-e
A "highly conserved" protein of influenza viruses.

Even in the face of such alluring theories the universal flu vaccine is still years away.

and Swedish scientists are attempting to produce a broad-spectrum vaccine. European scientists are calling their effort the Universal Vaccine Project. Animal studies conducted by Dutch researchers at the Flanders Interuniversity Institute for Biotechnology in Gent demonstrated that a vaccine targeting M2-e can be protective. After immunizing mice with a vaccine that targeted M2-e, the animals were exposed to flu viruses potent enough to kill them. The mice survived. Scientists are optimistic that a universal vaccine ultimately could provide long-term protection for humans.

27. Many groups oppose vaccines. Is the flu vaccine among them?

Despite the good vaccines can do, the issue of vaccination remains highly charged. Numerous consumer groups have marshaled against vaccinations, including the flu vaccine, blaming the preparations for a wide range of ills. Autism spectrum disorders are high on the list of childhood disorders that some parents have linked to vaccines. Federal health officials insist there is no link between autism and vaccines.

The National Vaccine Information Center, founded by Barbara Loe Fisher, is a Virginia-based organization that has taken the public health community to task, claiming vaccines do more harm than good.

The center keeps readers of its Web site apprised of anti-vaccine activities and provides information on what it believes are the ill effects caused by vaccines. The center's opposition encompasses a wide spectrum of vaccine preparations, from those against common childhood illnesses to Gardasil (quadrivalent human papillomavirus recombinant vaccine), the cervical cancer vaccine. The group is opposed to annual flu vaccinations for babies and children, citing a report from the *British Medical Journal* in 2006 that declared vaccines had not been fully studied. Infectious disease experts at CDC and WHO have argued strongly against the study's findings.

28. Are there groups in favor of immunizing children against influenza?

In addition to major government health agencies, such as the CDC, the National Institute of Allergy and Infectious Diseases, and all state and local health agencies in each of the 50 states, the American Academy of Pediatrics, the American Academy of Family Physicians, the American Public Health Association, and the Infectious Diseases Society of America support vaccinating children against the flu. These are just a few of the major agencies and organizations that either have policies or have issued statements favoring flu vaccination for children.

Immunizing children against influenza also is supported by a network of parents and pediatricians who belong to a non-profit organization known as Families Fighting Flu, Inc. The membership is composed of people who've experienced the death of a child or whose child developed severe complications as a result of the flu. The membership works vigorously to improve rates of pediatric flu vaccination nationwide.

Campaigning to encourage the unvaccinated to be immunized against influenza, even if it's late November or getting close to the end of the year, is a role Families Fighting Flu has played in the larger public health community. The organization also provides a support network for parents who experience a flu-related tragedy. Dr. Julie Gerberding of the CDC has spoken on the organization's behalf to underscore influenza's seriousness.

PART THREE

Antiviral Medications

What is drug resistance?
Does it occur only with flu medications?

What is a virus, and what should I know about
the influenza virus?

I heard that with a single sneeze or cough, a flu virus
can remain suspended and viable at ceiling height for
nearly 20 minutes as it drifts to the floor.
Is this true?

More . . .

29. What are antiviral medications?

For more than a quarter century, doctors have turned to a class of medications called antivirals to help fight influenza. Antivirals are an important component in your healthcare provider's arsenal because they stop the virus from replicating. With that said, antivirals are not a replacement for vaccination and should not be used in place of flu vaccines. As vital as the medications are to public health, they are not perfect. There are noteworthy side effects and serious concerns about drug resistance.

The drugs can be used in one of two ways: as treatment for influenza, or as a preventive (**chemoprophylaxis**) to stop the infection before it starts. Studies have shown that any one of the approved antiviral medications can reduce the amount of time you are sick with the flu if the drugs are taken within the first 2 days of the onset of symptoms.

Four antiviral medications have been approved in the United States by the Food and Drug Administration. They are **amantadine (Symmetrel); rimantadine (Flumadine); zanamivir (Relenza), and oseltamivir (Tamiflu).** Of the four, only oseltamivir has been researched as a preventive. It is a component in the Strategic National Stockpile and is to be administered in the event of a major flu emergency. As with all of the stockpile's contents, federal health officials have already developed strict guidelines governing how the doses are to be distributed.

Amantadine and rimantadine, which are not in the federal stockpile, belong to the class of antiviral medications called the **adamantanes**. These drugs are only effective against Type A influenza and help stop a flu infection by targeting hemagglutinin, H, the flu virus surface protein. H is needed for a flu virus to attach to a host's cells. Amantadine and rimantadine were designed to prevent viruses from attaching and setting off the cascade of events that lead to the infection of additional cells in the lungs.

Zanamivir and oseltamivir are effective against Types A and B and zero in on the flu viral protein known as neuraminidase, or N. Because their target is neuraminidase, these drugs are known as neuraminidase inhibitors. They block N, which is an enzyme that flu viruses use to break free from a cell after infection.

Amantadine, the oldest of the four, was approved by the FDA in 1976. Federal regulators approved rimantadine in 1993. The neuraminidase inhibitors were approved in 1999. In addition to these four drugs, pharmaceutical companies are actively working on the development of others.

Antiviral medications have been prescribed to blunt the effects of influenza in a number of situations. They have been useful in nursing homes and other long-term care facilities where people 65 years and older are particularly vulnerable. The medications also have been especially useful on cruise ships where outbreaks—unless controlled—can spread quickly among crew members and passengers. When onboard health-care providers receive positive results from tests revealing that someone on the ship has the flu, an antiviral can then be prescribed to prevent an outbreak. Only oseltamivir has been fully tested as a flu preventive.

Antiviral drugs are useful in stopping the spread of influenza in homes with newborns too young to be vaccinated. Parents or other household members who may have been exposed to the flu can take an antiviral medication to block transmitting influenza to the baby. In addition to these instances, antivirals also have been used with some success in the treatment of patients who have been hospitalized for bird flu.

But even with the benefits antiviral drugs offer, they pose a number of serious health issues. They produce side effects. Flu viruses can develop resistance to them, and when preventing

admantane

A class of antiviral medications capable of relieving flu symptoms. The two drugs in this case are amantadine (Symmetrel) and rimantadine (Flumadine).

Antiviral Medications

influenza is the aim, the drug must be prescribed within a certain critical time frame. In 2005, Dr. Rick Bright, then a research scientist at the CDC, found in a startling study that influenza A viruses had been developing resistance to amantadine and rimantadine for years. Resistance refers to the capacity of flu viruses to thwart medications, essentially rendering antiviral drugs useless.

Bright's study revealed a 12% increase in resistance to the two drugs since the mid-1990s. The resistance remained persistent, and the following year, Dr. Julie Gerberding, the agency's director, declared an indefinite embargo on the drugs and asked doctors not to prescribe them until there was evidence that flu viruses were again susceptible to defeat by amantadine and rimantadine. Apparently, circulating flu viruses remained defiantly resistant because more than a year after Dr. Gerberding's announcement, the embargo was still in effect.

There are issues involving zanamivir and oseltamivir as well. Zanamivir is not simple to take and must be inhaled, as a mist from a device. Patients with asthma and lung disorders can develop spasms and are advised to use the medication with caution. Even though side effects are minimal in most patients, a 2001 study in Great Britain found that elderly patients could not easily use the inhalation device, which made the medication less useful for them. However, studies since that time have not shown the same problem, which means that older patients probably fare as well as younger ones prescribed zanamivir.

The FDA issued a warning in 2006 about oseltamivir's potential to cause unusual behavioral problems in children. The warning grew out of observations of children in Japan who had been prescribed the medication but were affected by serious psychological side effects. Unusual behavior ranged from hallucinations and delirium to suicidal tendencies. FDA health officials recommended that these problems be noted on the oseltamivir label and that close monitoring of children taking the medication is vital. Two years before the behavior problems were revealed, many people had begun hoarding oseltamivir out of fear that a pandemic was imminent. Oseltamivir hoarding was reminiscent of similar hoarding of ciprofloxacin (Cipro), an antibiotic that was in the spotlight during the anthrax scare in the fall of 2001.

30. Couldn't I simply take a pill rather than get a flu shot?

Although it seems infinitely simpler, not to mention less painful to swallow a pill than it is to get a shot, antiviral medications are not an easy solution to avoiding the flu. Getting an annual jab in the upper arm—or a quick vaccine spray in your nostril—is still the preferred way to prevent the flu. Antiviral medications have to be prescribed and taken with care. As mentioned in Question 29, flu viruses are very crafty when it comes to medications and can develop resistance to the drugs that are designed to destroy them. When too many people take antiviral medications, viruses have more opportunity to be exposed to them and develop the capacity to repel them.

31. What is drug resistance? Does it occur only with flu medications?

Drug resistance is one of the most serious medical problems today, and it is seen across a vast number of organisms— bacteria, viruses, protozoa, and mycoplasma. Drug-resistant strains are able to adapt and even thrive in the presence of potent medications. The frightening aspect of drug resistance is that some organisms are capable of repelling more than one drug, which in effect makes them **multidrug resistant**. In such instances, healthcare providers have even fewer options for sick patients. CDC and WHO health officials are concerned about the fierce resistance Type A flu viruses have shown to the adamantane class of medications, amantadine

multidrug resistant

When a disease-causing organism is able to resist distinct drugs or chemicals of a wide variety of structure and function targeted at eradicating the organism.

and rimantadine. Drug-resistant flu viruses now join the ranks of other highly infectious organisms that are capable of multiplying in the presence of once-powerful medications.

Exactly how the Type A flu viruses became resistant to the adamantanes is a matter of debate. For example, when Dr. Gerberding announced the resistance problem in 2006, she also acknowledged being puzzled as to how the resistance became so pervasive. Perhaps it was the result of a mutation in H3N2 flu viruses (the predominant strain that circulates in flu season); or it could have been the result of an overuse of the adamantanes in parts of the world where the drugs are widely used in the poultry industry and purchased indiscriminately by individuals over the counter.

Although some medical ethicists have cautioned that it is not in the interest of global cooperation to point fingers at certain healthcare practices in some countries, others have called for open discussions on how to use the drugs most judiciously. In many parts of Asia, for example, the adamantanes can be purchased in stores the way people in the United States and Canada can buy simple headache remedies. When potent antivirals are so easily accessible and used without prescription, they eventually have less impact.

Without a prescription and direction from a healthcare provider, people may not take enough medication to eliminate an infection. Some individuals might take a drug long enough to feel better. This could mean that an antiviral was taken long enough to destroy weaker viruses but that hardier ones remain behind—and are still transmissible. Hardier viruses, like their weaker counterparts, were exposed to the medication. The difference is that hardier viruses were not affected. When this scenario is repeated by thousands of individuals who've all taken the same drug, the result is hardier drug-resistant strains becoming persistent in the population. With only hardy, drug-repelling strains in circulation, the medications can become powerless. As infections spread, there is nothing available for healthcare providers to use to stop transmission.

The U.S. embargo on amantadine and rimantadine has been one solution to resistance. When the drug pressure is off the viruses, it is more likely that strains in circulation ultimately will become susceptible to the antivirals. Precisely how long that will take remains an unanswered question.

32. Can drug-resistant flu viruses spread around the world?

Just as nonresistant flu viruses can spread around the world in endless chains of coughing, sneezing, shaking hands, and other forms of close contact, so too can drug-resistant strains. One of the greatest fears of public health authorities worldwide is the spread of drug-resistant influenza strains in a major influenza outbreak. Infections become more difficult to treat and control because drugs that once defeated the microbes are no longer effective. Public health officials say it is important that people learn about drug resistance and the need to avoid using powerful antivirals and antibiotics when they do not need them. Discriminate use of the medications, they say, helps keep drug-resistant strains out of circulation.

33. What is a virus?

A virus is one of the smallest infectious entities known to biologists.

As simple as that may seem, it is probably difficult to picture and, admittedly, is somewhat difficult to explain. The challenge here is conveying the notion of how incredibly small viruses actually are. Some scientists prefer to draw upon illustrations of *largest* and *smallest* to define how imperceptibly tiny the concept of *small* can actually be.

A virus is one of the smallest infectious entities known to biologists.

Two decades ago in a classic text titled *Viruses,* renowned virologist Dr. Arthur J. Levine wrote that for centuries people have been fascinated with concepts of largest and smallest. For mathematicians, he says, the notions of largest and smallest are best understood in a comparison between infinity and zero. For physicists, he defines that juxtaposition as the vastness of an ever-expanding universe opposite the imponderable smallness of particles tinier than atoms.

For biologists, Levine muses there is respect for the grandeur of whales and redwood trees and equal respect for the awesome power of the entities at the opposite end of the size spectrum: viruses. Viruses are unique in nature for a variety of reasons, not just their infinitesimal size. Viruses are neither living nor dead. They are the ultimate parasites that exist at a difficult-to-imagine juncture between the living and nonliving. And because they are parasitic, they require a host's cells to replicate. Yet the influenza virus is made up of only eight genes swathed in a protein coat. As simple as that sounds, flu viruses are capable of serious—and sometimes breathtaking—consequences.

Viruses are neither living nor dead.

34. Do flu viruses infect all cells or only certain cells?

Like most viruses, those that cause influenza are highly specific with a preference for only a certain kind of cell. In the case of waterfowl, the original hosts of flu viruses, the preferred cells are those in the intestinal tract. In humans and other mammals, flu viruses have an affinity for the respiratory system, homing in on the lungs. Pigs and ferrets, for example, develop a disease that is virtually identical to that experienced by people.

To get a better idea of viral specificity, it is perhaps a good idea to develop an understanding of other types of viruses and the cells they prefer. Many types of viruses have specificity for a certain kind of cell in the body to which it latches on and then invades. The human immunodeficiency virus, which causes AIDS, has a preference for the immune system cell known as the CD-4 lymphocyte. Herpes viruses home in on nerve cells. Hepatitis viruses prefer liver cells. The poliovirus, which once caused frightening waves of crippling disease worldwide, zeroes in on cells in the human intestinal tract.

But even with all that scientists have learned about influenza viruses, where they originate and how they are transmitted annually around the world, influenza viruses still pose numerous research questions. One, of course, is probing how potentially deadly avian strains can undergo certain genetic transformations to become threats to human populations.

35. What should I know about the influenza virus?

As mentioned earlier, there are three types of influenza viruses: A, B, and C. Despite differences, all belong to the viral family known as *Orthomyxoviridae.* Interestingly, the closest relatives to this family are not the viruses of the common cold, but those responsible for mumps and measles. Probably more than a few people would think that with the multitude of common cold viruses, possibly 200 or more, a few of the pathogens would show some kind of kinship to influenza. After all, the symptoms produced by mumps and measles are nothing like those of influenza whereas the symptoms of the flu and the common cold are much more alike. Yet as logical as that may seem, virologists emphasize that it is not the outward effects of an infection that relate one viral family to another, but the specific genetic characteristics of the microbes.

The common cold can be triggered by any of the viruses belonging to three broad families: **adenoviruses**, coronaviruses, and rhinoviruses. These three types of viruses package their genetic information in strands of DNA. Flu viruses, and those that cause mumps and rubeola (measles), package theirs in the genetic material known as RNA.

Orthomyxoviridae

A family of RNA viruses that include five genera: Influenzavirus A, Influenzavirus B, Influenzavirus C, Thogotovirus, and Isavirus.

adenoviruses

A family of about 40 DNA viruses known to cause human infections, including the common cold.

You are capable of infecting others at least a day before you start feeling any symptoms and up to a full week after you've become ill.

Here is something else you might find interesting about the pathogens that cause influenza: You are capable of infecting others at least a day before you start feeling any symptoms and up to a full week after you've become ill. Even though the flu vaccine is a public health tool of great importance, on many occasions, simple hygiene can help prevent you from spreading your infection to others. Old-fashioned hygiene also can protect you from catching flu viruses from someone else. These measures include frequent hand washing with plenty of soap and warm water. Washing long enough to sing the song "Happy Birthday to You" twice is usually enough time to ensure that you have thoroughly cleaned your hands. You should always cover your mouth when coughing, and you should wash your hands immediately afterward. When possible try to stay clear of people who are sick. However, that bit of advice may be difficult to follow if you are the parent of a family member, especially a young child or have an elderly parent, who requires your help. Another hygiene tip to help prevent infection with influenza viruses is to avoid rubbing your eyes or touching your nose and mouth. If your hands are contaminated, you can easily infect yourself.

36. The avian flu virus is referred to as H5N1, and the seasonal flu virus as H3N2. What do those letters and numbers stand for?

As mentioned earlier, H stands for hemagglutinin and N for neuraminidase, two proteins on the surface of the flu virus. Each protein plays a role in the infection process. You may recall from earlier in the discussion that a flu virus looks like a mace, the medieval weapon noted for its spikes. The virus uses H to latch on and enter a host's cells. Once the host's genes have been commandeered and scores of new viruses have been produced inside a cell, the pathogens use N to break out of the cell. They emerge as fully formed new viruses free to invade other cells in your lungs and begin the rapid replication process all over again.

To understand what the combination of H and N means with respect to individual viruses, you may recall from earlier in the discussion that each influenza A virus has different combinations of these two proteins. Virologists have determined that there are 16 possible H variations and 9 possible for N. For example, the strain of bird flu that has raised concerns around the world has a number 5 subtype of H and a number 1 subtype of N. That is why the deadly pathogen is known as H5N1. Only avian viruses with subtypes H5 or H7 are known to cause the highly pathogenic form of influenza. Seasonal flu is usually designated H3N2 or H1N1.

37. I heard that with a single sneeze or cough, a flu virus can remain suspended and viable at ceiling height for nearly 20 minutes as it drifts to the floor. Is this true?

True it is. The influenza virus is extraordinarily hardy. It can remain viable and infectious while suspended. It also remains viable for more than half an hour on a variety of common surfaces. Tabletops, countertops, plastic and metal doorknobs and handles—virtually any surface that someone infected with the virus might touch.

38. Why is the inhaled vaccine referred to as "live but weakened"?

The reference is merely one way to convey an important point: The virus is in a crippled and noninfectious state and as such is incapable of causing the flu. The appropriate term, as mentioned in Question 15, is attenuated. Using the word live is a simple, though somewhat inaccurate way of noting viral status. By the same token, using the word killed to denote the status of flu viruses contained in injected vaccines also is inaccurate even though it sounds quite reassuring. To be more precise, you might want to think of those viruses as inactivated. Using words such as live, killed, or dead with respect to viruses is meant to convey to the public that attenuated and inactivated viruses pose no harm.

39. You mentioned that waterfowl are a natural reservoir for influenza viruses. What about mammals? Do dogs, cats, and pigs also catch the flu? Are they passing the same viruses back and forth?

Virtually all mammalian species catch the flu. Ferrets are not only susceptible, they serve in laboratories as models of human infection. Ferrets exhibit the same respiratory symptoms as people when they catch the flu, but they are not the only members of the animal kingdom vulnerable to influenza.

For instance, concern arose in 2004 with anecdotal reports in Thailand of domestic cats exposed to birds with the H5N1 avian influenza strain. The reports were startling because scientists previously believed that cats were resistant to influenza A viruses, the type to which H5N1 belongs. Experiments conducted at Erasmus University in the Netherlands confirmed the Thai anecdotes, adding to the fear that domestic animals in close contact with sick birds may not only catch the disease but ultimately can pass it along to humans.

Domestic cats have not been the only felines in Thailand to catch H5N1. When zookeepers in Bangkok reported serious respiratory illnesses in tigers, scientists again were surprised to find infection with H5N1, the bird flu strain. Leopards in Thailand also were stricken with it. Tracing a probable cause, zookeepers found that some of the large cats had eaten chickens infected with the deadly virus. Additional studies found that tigers not only caught avian influenza, they were also able to pass the infection to tigers that had not eaten tainted birds.

Scientists also find other instances of cross-species infection instructive. Teams of researchers worldwide are investigating how flu viruses that are common in one species make the leap to another. Once a virus that routinely circulates in one species jumps to another, the pathogen accomplishes an important step in the evolution of an outbreak, experts say.

Attention has been focused on pigs for many years because they can be infected with avian, human, and swine influenza viruses at the same time. All of these viruses can reassort—swap genes—in pigs, leading to new strains that can be passed into the human population. The swine flu scare of 1976 was based on notions of gene swapping that public health experts thought would lead to a major human outbreak. Fear heightened when soldiers started getting sick.

At Fort Dix, New Jersey, where a few hundred soldiers were infected with swine flu, at least four developed pneumonia as a consequence. A fifth of the soldiers died. Military health officials thought the flu, fueled by the animal strain, would spread beyond Fort Dix and cause waves of severe infections in the general population. A sweeping outbreak, driven by a swine flu virus, never materialized. More extensive studies following the national panic revealed the virus had been circulating in the general population for years but had caused only mild illness in those who contracted it.

In more recent years, the Centers for Disease Control and Prevention reported that H3N8, a strain commonly seen in horses, crossed species to infect dogs, leading to a serious flu outbreak in canines. In 2005, the flu swept relentlessly through kennels and dog-grooming establishments, causing runny noses and triggering coughs and fevers as high as 106° Fahrenheit. The severity of the outbreak occurred largely because dogs had never been exposed to the virus, so were completely without immunity. Greyhounds in Florida were among the first to be infected in an outbreak that quickly spread to virtually all breeds of dogs. An estimated 20,000 racing greyhounds died of the flu at 20 tracks in seven states.

More extensive studies following the national panic surrounding the swine flu revealed the virus had been circulating in the general population for years but had caused only mild illness in those who contracted it.

Dr. Cynda Crawford, a veterinary research scientist at the University of Florida, reported about the leap of H3N8 from horses to dogs in the journal *Science* and during a CDC-sponsored news conference. She said the virus spread most efficiently among dogs housed in close quarters. But the strain was so virulent that studies eventually showed H3N8 could be transmitted from dog to dog as they passed each other on the street.

The flu outbreak triggered by H3N8 offered an important lesson, Crawford and other researchers underscored, because it revealed that once a virus leaps to a new species, it can spread efficiently. H3N8 is firmly established in the dog population. Prior to the 2005 outbreak scientists knew of the virus for 40 years, but only as a cause of influenza in horses. What remains unclear is exactly how and when the virus jumped the species barrier from horses to dogs.

40. Why do so many influenza viruses originate in China? Is there a link to animal species?

Earlier it was explained that flu strains destined to become significant causes of infection can begin anywhere in the world—and they do. But there has been a very strong Asian link, particularly to China. Scientists have long theorized that not only have many flu strains over the last 3,000 to 4,000 years originated in China, the vast proportion are probably associated with the country's farming practices. For centuries, Chinese farmers have raised ducks and pigs in close proximity, often within the same pens where the two species have nudged each other for food and space. Dozens upon dozens of these farms adjoin each other over thousands of acres throughout China's countryside. In addition, domestic ducks tend to roam in search of food and therefore have ample opportunity to come in contact with infected migratory birds—wild ducks and geese—that temporarily arrive on the farms to swipe food from their domesticated kin.

As wild birds resume their journey, they leave behind virus-laden urine and feces, which can easily infect domesticated fowl. The United Nations estimates that 80% of the world's domestic duck population resides on backyard farms in China and Vietnam, which probably helps explain why many of the initial human infections involving avian flu occurred in those countries.

Domestic birds, meanwhile, can pass influenza viruses to pigs. Because ducks and pigs are in such close contact, their pens become living laboratories for flu transmission. A theory known as "the **mixing vessel**" suggests that when pigs contract flu viruses from ducks, gene swapping occurs within the pig. Swine possess genetic factors that render avian flu viruses more amenable to transmission among mammals, including humans. Scientists have strongly suggested that Chinese farmers are likely the first to catch the flu in a global chain of flu infections. This scenario has been suggested as a model for seasonal flu strains.

> **mixing vessel**
> A theory explaining how flu viruses from different species might combine in one animal to produce a novel virus.

But there is still concern that pigs might serve as a mixing vessel for a deadlier strain, such as H5N1, providing it with the necessary genetic changes to make it easily transmissible from person to person. Most outbreaks of H5N1 have occurred on small-scale farms. The United Nations reports that farmers who sell their fowl for a living often do so through live-bird markets that "bring different species together in usually unsanitary conditions," furthering the possibilities for flu transmission.

41. Why don't wild waterfowl get sick from the flu viruses they carry?

Scientists at the World Health Organization suggest that waterfowl probably have carried flu viruses for centuries and have not been harmed. Because of such long-term adaptation, the influenza strains that inhabit the birds' intestines probably will never prove lethal to them. Looking at it another way, the viral strains are as natural to the birds' intestinal tracts as are the bacteria that thrive in the guts of mammals. Flu viruses, therefore, have ample opportunity to multiply in aquatic birds. H5N1, the avian influenza strain that has captured the most attention in recent years, is not the only virus that is pathogenic to people. Scientists also have isolated H7N7 and H9N2. Possibly others have yet to be identified.

Millions of waterfowl traverse global distances across migratory flyways, the vast "freeways in the sky." These are pathways that migratory birds know instinctively and travel seasonally. Maps of the flyways, which have been drawn for the United Nations, show vast looping and zig-zag patterns that take flocks along migratory paths that circumnavigate the globe.

PART FOUR

Influenza and Children

How vulnerable are children to
seasonal flu?

Are childhood influenza vaccines identical to the ones
given to adults?

What's the point of vaccinating your child against
one respiratory illness when there are others out there
that are equally as serious?

More . . .

42. How vulnerable are children to seasonal flu?

Rates of influenza infection are highest among children, and this underscores why the Centers for Disease Control and Prevention expanded the range of ages that it recommends for annual flu vaccinations. For years the Advisory Committee on Immunization Practices, the panel that counsels the CDC on vaccine policies, recommended that babies from the age of 6 months through 23 months receive the vaccine. But in 2006 the panel expanded its recommendation, advising that healthy children between 6 months and 5 years be vaccinated annually. In 2008, the CDC panel went even further, recommending flu vaccination for all healthy children between the ages of 6 months and 18 years. (Apart from these recommendations the CDC has had longstanding vaccination guidelines for children with respiratory and immune-compromising conditions.)

Expanding the range of ages eligible for the vaccine was important for a variety of reasons. Children not only are frequent carriers of the flu virus, they often live in households with infant siblings and/or elderly grandparents. Moreover, the National Foundation for Infectious Diseases indicates that babies younger than 24 months "are hospitalized with influenza-related complications at rates similar to those of people 65 years and older."

For children under the age of 15 years old, every 6 to 15 hospitalizations are attributable to influenza when flu viruses are in circulation, according to the National Foundation for Infectious Diseases. Also, federal statistics demonstrate that children between 6 months and 5 years have higher rates of flu-related visits to clinics and emergency rooms compared with visits for other illnesses. High-risk children, those with respiratory or immune-compromising conditions, are five times more likely than healthy children of the same age to be hospitalized for complications related to the flu.

When the 2003 flu season struck especially early—cases were being reported in September—children were particularly hard hit. It is also important to note the major strain in circulation, A-Fujian. It caused serious illness, which led to hospitalizations of children from toddlers to teens throughout the United States. Forty state health agencies later confirmed 153 deaths as flu-related in the 2003–2004 influenza season.

In an analysis published in the *New England Journal of Medicine* in December 2005 that summarized the outbreak's effects among children, epidemiologists from the CDC led by Drs. Niranjan Bhat and Jennifer G. Wright concluded that the median age of infections was 3 years old. Forty-seven children died outside a hospital setting, and 45 died within 3 days of the infection's onset. Bacterial co-infections were identified in 24 cases. But epidemiologists found that even though 47% of the children had been healthy prior to influenza infection, the majority either had an underlying condition recognized to increase the risk of influenza-related complications or some other chronic condition that weakened their ability to fight the flu. Scientists who conducted the research concluded: "High priority should be given to improvements in influenza-vaccine coverage and improvements in the diagnosis and treatment of influenza to reduce childhood mortality from infection."

43. What are the complications of influenza in children?

First and foremost, the majority of children who catch the flu are miserable for a few days but are back on the soccer field or in ballet class in no time—as if an illness never occurred. There are, however, numerous ways in which the flu can lead to secondary problems, which is why flu vaccination can help children avoid more than one illness. Children are more likely than adults to have stomach upset and diarrhea as part of a flu infection. Additional complications can include ear and/or sinus infections and, worse still, bacterial pneumonia. In some rare instances, children may develop a condition known as Reye's syndrome, a serious disorder marked by nausea, vomiting, lethargy, irregular breathing, and in some cases, delirium. The condition is extraordinarily rare, affecting 0.1 children per 100,000 in the U.S. population.

44. Can you provide further information about Reye's syndrome and explain its link to aspirin and the flu?

Children on long-term aspirin therapy (i.e., patients with rheumatoid arthritis) are at elevated risk of contracting Reye's syndrome if they catch the flu because the syndrome tends to strike after a viral illness and particularly among children who have taken aspirin or similar medications. Healthcare providers have long highlighted the importance of flu vaccination for children on long-term aspirin treatment.

The National Reye's Syndrome Foundation describes the condition as one that can strike swiftly, attacking all organ systems, especially the brain and liver. Even though a cause and a cure remain elusive, research has established a link between the use of aspirin and other salicylate-containing medications. The medications have been statistically linked to the syndrome. There are no scientific data showing how the medications are involved in the disease. To remain on the safe side, doctors say aspirin should not be given to children experiencing a viral illness, such as the flu.

Studies also have shown that Reye's syndrome is more prevalent in the population when viral diseases reach epidemic proportions. Severe influenza B outbreaks have been followed by an upsurge in Reye's syndrome cases, for example. Reye's syndrome primarily is seen among youngsters between the ages of 4 and 16 years old.

Influenza and Children

45. Are parents and doctors heeding vaccination recommendations?

Despite the importance—and urgency—that public health authorities have attached to childhood flu vaccination, a growing body of research suggests that many children are going without annual flu protection. In an October 2006 report, the National Foundation for Infectious Diseases found that more than 8 million children with asthma should receive influenza vaccinations annually, but nearly 70% of children in this population were not receiving flu shots. The result is the lowest vaccination rate for any recommended childhood vaccine in the United States.

Dr. Mary Patricia Norwalk, an epidemiologist at the University of Pittsburgh, similarly found in a survey of high-risk children that few were receiving annual flu shots. Her research was reported in 2006 in the *Journal of Urban Health*, a publication of the New York Academy of Medicine in New York City. The academy has long focused on a variety of health issues facing children, especially children from medically underserved communities throughout the United States.

46. Does a pervasive fear of vaccines prevent some parents from having their children vaccinated?

Many parents who avoid vaccinating their children would not say that they fear vaccines, but that they believe vaccines have not been sufficiently studied in children. Many anti-vaccination organizations cite references—usually their own—to support claims that vaccines are dangerous and should not be given to children. They claim that giving multiple vaccines at one time, a common practice in pediatric health care, is particularly dangerous. They also raise concerns about giving vaccines that contain mercury-based thimerosal, a vaccine additive used as a preservative in some but not all vaccines.

Since 2001, most vaccines manufactured for pediatric use in the United States have not contained thimerosal or contain only trace amounts. The U.S. Food and Drug Administration estimates the trace amounts of thimerosal to be less than 1 microgram of mercury per dose. Manufacturers also have switched from multidose vials for certain childhood vaccines because these types of injectables require use of the preservative. In recent years, manufacturers of flu vaccines have produced about nine million thimerosal-free doses for pediatric use. As mentioned earlier, anti-vaccination groups contend that vaccines can cause autism and other devastating neurologic and autoimmune disorders. Scientists have not corroborated those claims.

Persistence of pro and con positions in the vaccine debate does not mean each side's evidence carries equal weight. Vaccination has existed as a public health practice in North America for more than two centuries, starting with the smallpox vaccine. Scientific evidence has demonstrated that childhood diseases (mumps, measles, and chickenpox) that once caused widespread morbidity in communities are no longer spread thanks to vaccination. Smallpox has disappeared from the planet; polio exists only in small pockets of the underdeveloped world. Diphtheria and whooping cough are very rarely diagnosed. Public health authorities do not contend that vaccines are perfect and free of all conceivable side effects, but that they are, on the whole, safe preventive measures whose benefits far outweigh their risks—and that view extends to the flu vaccine.

herd immunity

Refers to the protection of a small minority of unvaccinated people because the majority of the population has been vaccinated against a contagious illness.

Looking at the anti-vaccine effort in another way, it is reasonable to argue that the movement has grown because activists live during an era largely free of the horrific diseases now prevented by vaccines. Some vaccine-preventable diseases have been nonexistent in the West for decades, others for more than a century. Anyone who remains unvaccinated in Western countries benefits from **herd immunity**.

This type of immunity occurs when a community's majority has been vaccinated and thus becomes incapable of catching and spreading certain infections. When millions of people have been vaccinated against, say, diphtheria, a highly contagious and potentially deadly bacterial disease, the infection cannot be transmitted, allowing the unvaccinated to benefit.

Diphtheria, which once killed millions of people, is reemerging in parts of the former Soviet Union and elsewhere in the world where vaccination efforts have not been on par with immunization strategies in the West. With global travel now simpler and more common, it is conceivable that a reemerging disease, such as diphtheria, can be transported to any city in the United States or Canada in a matter of hours. Herd immunity would not be possible if the disease were to spread among the unvaccinated.

Although it is tempting to refer to the information promoted by the anti-vaccine movement as irrational fears based on junk science, it is important to take note of the sincerity with which the activists base their opposition and their strong concerns about thimerosal. Many avoid vaccination out of the strong belief that vaccines will do more harm than good for their children.

47. Are childhood influenza vaccines identical to the ones given to adults?

There are *slight* differences between the flu vaccines administered to adults and those offered to children. Adults receive what is known as a whole virus vaccine; children receive a split-virus vaccine. And there are also some differences in how the shots are administered in some instances. Children between the ages of 6 months and 9 years old who are receiving a flu shot for the first time need two vaccine doses. Preferably, the first dose is given in September and is followed

Adults receive what is known as a whole virus vaccine; children receive a split-virus vaccine. And there are also some differences in how the shots are administered in some instances.

by a second dose 28 days later. According to the Centers for Disease Control and Prevention, the first dose "primes" the immune system whereas the second dose provides immune protection. As with adults, it takes about 2 weeks for a child to achieve full immunity from vaccination.

48. Isn't it useless to vaccinate a child against the flu when schools are overflowing with children carrying cold and flu viruses, especially during winter months?

Why risk the flu when you don't have to? Vaccination can help prevent an illness that sometimes carries serious consequences. U.S. federal health authorities estimate that 20,000 children in the United States are hospitalized annually for flu complications. Although the CDC strongly recommends flu vaccinations for children between the ages of 6 months and 18 years, annual shots for healthy children and teens older than 5 are still at the discretion of parents. There are, however, several notable exceptions.

Government health authorities strongly recommend influenza vaccination for children between the ages of 5 and 18 years when the youngster has asthma or other pulmonary problems; suffers from chronic heart or kidney conditions; has diabetes, sickle cell anemia, or any condition that suppresses immunity. Vaccination is not recommended for children who are allergic to eggs. You may recall from earlier in the discussion that eggs are a necessary component in the vaccine manufacturing process.

Parents can ask their healthcare provider whether the vaccine offered to their child is free of thimerosal, the preservative added to the preparations. Some children have had allergic reactions to thimerosal, which is also added to contact lens solution. Thimerosal is a controversial substance because some parents have linked it to autism and other devastating conditions. In the United States and Canada, millions of vaccines marked for pediatric use are thimerosal-free. But it is probably a good idea to check, especially if you have strong concerns about the compound.

49. Our baby contracted respiratory syncytial virus, and the symptoms are identical to influenza. What's the point of vaccinating your child against one respiratory illness when there are others out there that are equally as serious?

Respiratory syncytial virus (RSV) causes a serious infection and is the most common cause of pneumonia and **bronchiolitis** in children under 12 months of age. Another common cause of pneumonia and bronchiolitis in babies is a virus called **parainfluenza virus**, which is explained in greater detail in Question 50. Initial signs of RSV infection are fever, cough, and runny nose, symptoms that easily can be mistaken for influenza or perhaps be mistakenly diagnosed by parents as the common cold. It is best that a healthcare provider examine any baby exhibiting respiratory symptoms so that a proper course of action can be pursued.

50. What is parainfluenza virus?

Parainfluenza virus refers to any of the four viral subtypes belonging to the *Paramyxovirus* family, all of which are capable of causing significant respiratory illnesses in babies and very young children. In older children, teens, and adults younger than 65, infection with any of the types of parainfluenza virus tends to cause only mild respiratory symptoms. Parainfluenza viral infection also can cause significant respiratory disease in people who are 65 or older. Viruses in the *Paramyxovirus* family rank high among those that cause respiratory illnesses in young children.

Respiratory syncytial virus (RSV)

A common virus that causes mild respiratory conditions in adults but can cause more serious conditions, such as bronchiolitis, croup, and pneumonia in infants and children.

bronchiolitis

Inflammation of the smallest air passages in the lungs, the bronchioles.

parainfluenza virus

A viral infection that causes bronchiolitis and is most often diagnosed in children.

Despite a name that suggests a relationship to influenza, this viral family does not cause the flu. One of the most significant conditions caused by a parainfluenza virus is croup. The disorder can be quite frightening for parents to observe, and many feel helpless as they try to comfort an affected child. Croup is typified by hoarseness and a coarse barking cough. Children run a fever and experience difficulty breathing. Those who have the worst symptoms usually are between the ages of 3 months and 5 years. As with influenza viral infection, parainfluenza virus is spread through aerosolized respiratory secretions or contact with contaminated surfaces or objects.

Scientists have identified four types of parainfluenza viruses, which are noteworthy for the respiratory conditions they cause, and essentially where the pathogens occur globally. Parainfluenza virus types 1, 2, and 3 are found worldwide, but type 4 has been identified only in the United States. Type 1 is the leading cause of croup, but the others, especially type 2, have been linked to the condition as well. Type 3 is of concern to healthcare providers worldwide because of its association with pneumonia. Type 3 also is linked to bronchitis and bronchiolitis. Of the four parainfluenza viruses, type 4 is the one diagnosed least often and also is the one associated with milder forms of infection.

For most children, the incubation period with a parainfluenza viral infection usually runs 1 to 7 days. Currently, there is neither a vaccine nor an antiviral drug available despite decades of scientific work to produce ways of better coping with parainfluenza disease. Antiviral medications that are routinely used to stave off influenza infection have no effect on the parainfluenza viruses. However, very active scientific work is under way to develop a vaccine against types 1 and 3.

51. How safe are oseltamivir and other flu drugs for children?

The U.S. Food and Drug Administration has investigated several disturbing reports, revealing that flu medications can cause abnormal behavior and even death in children and teens. The reports first surfaced in Japan where hospitalized children were being treated for influenza. In 2005, about a dozen Japanese children died while taking oseltamivir, and at least one committed suicide. Self-injurious behavior surfaced while the youngster was being treated for influenza.

In March 2007, medical authorities in Japan ruled against prescribing the drug to anyone between the ages of 10 and 19 after more than 100 children and teens who were prescribed the medication exhibited signs of abnormal behavior. Japanese authorities then expanded their investigation to include stiff warnings for zanamivir, another influenza medication. According to an extensive study in Japan, some children who had taken zanamivir experienced hallucinations and delirium. The FDA has approved a stiff warning to be included on oseltamivir's label, urging close monitoring of children who are prescribed the drug. The agency began an investigation of zanamivir in 2007.

Nearly 50 million people worldwide have taken oseltamivir, including 21 million children, since its approval in 1999. Zanamivir has been prescribed to about 4 million people since it was first marketed the same year. U.S. health authorities underscore that despite the problems, influenza drugs are used differently in Japan. Why psychiatric problems and deaths started surfacing nearly a decade after the licensing of both drugs has not yet been explained. Throughout North America and elsewhere in the West, doctors have long emphasized the importance of vaccination, prescribing the medications only as a last resort.

Influenza and Children

PART FIVE

Influenza and Seniors, 65 Years and Older

As a senior, what should I know about my immune system?

What can be done about boosting the effectiveness of flu shots for older people?

Why are complications a concern in older people? What are some of the secondary illnesses that can occur as a result of influenza?

More . . .

52. My wife and I are in our 70s and we heard on the news that flu vaccination doesn't do much good for people our age. Why should we bother getting a shot?

As mentioned in Question 19, flu vaccination is not always 100% effective for people of any age, and it may not always prevent infection in people whose immunity has declined naturally with age. That said, research has shown that when seniors are vaccinated against the flu, the likelihood of hospitalization for flu-related complications is reduced by up to 70%. Even when the vaccine does not help prevent the infection, it does lessen its severity by shortening a bout with the flu.

For anyone confined to a nursing home or other long-term care facility, flu-related death is reduced by 80% among those who are vaccinated. Confined seniors are vulnerable to influenza because they are in a facility with numerous other people, which raises the likelihood of viral transmission. The situation is not unlike that of schools, dormitories, or other facilities where a significant number of people congregate.

The only factors that should dissuade you from getting a flu shot are allergies to the vaccine. Influenza can prove to be a particularly nasty respiratory infection in people 65 and older and is a significant cause of hospitalization and death. Of the estimated 36,000 annual flu deaths, the majority are people 65 and older.

Still, it is easy to understand why some seniors are confused about influenza vaccinations.

A study published in the *Archives of Internal Medicine* and reported widely by the news media a few years ago seemed to suggest that flu shots were useless for seniors. The U.S. government-funded analysis examined influenza vaccination data over a three-decade period and concluded that flu shots have not been as effective as they could have been in saving the lives of people in this age group.

But Dr. Lone Simonsen, the study's lead investigator, underscored that older people should not misinterpret the data. The study does not mean seniors should abandon the autumn vaccination ritual. She proposes, instead, that vaccine developers and policymakers rethink the vaccine. Better vaccines are needed to provide stronger protection, especially for frail individuals who are susceptible to infection and who are also very likely to be encumbered by other medical conditions.

Additional research by another team of medical investigators supports Simonsen's hypothesis. Researchers at the Veterans Administration Medical Center in Minneapolis found in a subsequent study that the annual vaccine reduces the risk of hospitalization and death in the elderly.

Dr. Kristin Nichol, chief of medicine at the VA, discovered after examining a decade's worth of data that flu vaccinations decreased hospitalizations for pneumonia by 27% and cut the overall death rate in half. The most eye-catching part of the research was her finding that flu vaccination helps reduce wintertime deaths for any reason, not just mortality related to influenza. Scientists refer to such deaths as "all-cause" mortality.

Nichol explained her findings for the Long Island newspaper *Newsday*: "What we know from other studies is that all-cause mortality spikes upward during flu season. These are deaths due to heart failure, cardiovascular disease and diabetes as well as other conditions."

But when people are vaccinated against influenza, she adds, deaths decline. Nichol theorizes that the flu might serve as an additional burden in unvaccinated people who are already encumbered by chronic conditions. Being unprotected from the flu might therefore lead to a higher death rate during winter when influenza viruses are in circulation.

Nichol and her colleagues studied thousands of people who belonged to health maintenance organizations throughout the United States. "We looked at the data by age, gender and whether they had frequent contacts with the health care system or very few contacts with the health care system. What we found were very clear benefits from vaccination."

53. Who transmits flu more readily, seniors or children?

Anyone can transmit the flu. However, studies repeatedly have shown that children and teenagers are more likely to catch the flu at school where many kids may be infected. As a result, youngsters can bring home the infection and pass it to family members, including vulnerable grandparents. Lone Simonsen, an epidemiologist at the National Institute of Allergy and Infectious Diseases who conducted a study on the effectiveness of influenza vaccination in the elderly (see Question 52), posited years ago that flu vaccination should be extended to include more children and teens. As mentioned earlier, in 2008 the CDC expanded the age group of children for whom it recommends annual flu vaccination. The CDC now advises that children between the ages of 23 months and 18 years are best served by a flu shot.

According to Simonsen and her colleagues, because school-age youngsters comprise the group most likely to transmit the flu virus, having a vaccination strategy that includes all school-age children through the age of 18 better serves the whole population, especially older people. Making school-age children the focus of a national vaccine program greatly reduces society's flu burden because those who transmit it most are guarded against infection.

Annual flu shots have been recommended for people 65 and older since the early 1960s. Changing the emphasis to focus vaccine policies on children and teens will likely have a greater impact on blunting flu transmission, many experts now believe.

54. As a senior, what should I know about my immune system?

The immune system is the body's surveillance and defense system that is on guard 24 hours 7 days a week to provide protection against myriad harmful invaders to which we are exposed daily. And it isn't just infectious agents that your immune system keeps at bay. Your immune system can help thwart the development of cancer, but that's another story. With age, immunity declines, and as a result, your body does not mount as vigorous a response as it did when you were younger. By the same token, the body does not respond as vigorously to vaccination. Some scientists refer to the phenomenon of decreased immunity as **immune senescence**.

immune senescence

An aging immune response.

Of course, the degree to which immunity declines depends on the individual. An extremely robust senior who is free of chronic conditions may be as healthy as someone decades younger and can produce a hardy immune response when vaccinated. When the population as a whole is taken into account, studies continually document that as people age, the capacity to fight infection is not as strong. Consequently, you are not only more vulnerable to the flu, you are also more likely to contract the secondary bacterial infections that can occur when the body is weakened by the influenza virus.

55. What are antibodies?

Whenever we are exposed to an infectious virus, we produce antibodies, tiny proteins that help repel infection. Antibodies are specific to each invading pathogen. Should the microbe be encountered again, the immune system recalls the previous infection and immediately releases antibodies already primed to deactivate the invader.

antibody

A Y-shaped protein that is made by the body's immune system in response to invasive foreign substances, such as bacteria, viruses, protozoa, fungi, toxins, and even transplanted organs.

Antibodies are produced by plasma cells, and are important components in the immune system's surveillance network. To deactivate an infectious virus an **antibody** must "bind" to a specific site on the virus. This site is known as an antigen. Antibodies are very important in the immune system's ability to remember previous infections. Even though public health officials recommend annual vaccination against influenza, the body does not completely forget encountering the flu virus in earlier years. During the great flu pandemic of 1918 when millions of young and otherwise hardy people died of the infection, scientists of the day happened upon a conundrum: Many healthy older people did not suffer as severe an illness. Why? Medical scientists now theorize that younger people apparently died of a highly aggressive immune response to the flu. Cells and proteins of the immune system ravaged the body in its attempt to destroy the virus. Healthy older people with a less reactive immune system were spared because their immune systems did not respond as aggressively to the pandemic strain. Of course, not all older people in that early-20th-century disaster survived the infection. But given that so many were able to pull through the most devastating flu season in history, scientists now posit that it's possible for healthy older people to survive a similar plague.

56. What can be done about boosting the effectiveness of flu shots for older people?

Many medical experts believe that flu vaccines tailored specifically for the elderly are what is needed to provide optimum defense against the flu. For such special vaccines to become a reality requires research based on what scientists know about the immunity of people as they age. Vaccines, you should understand, do not provide protection by themselves. Vaccines rely on the immune system to fight infectious diseases. The vaccine itself does not fight disease—your body does. It might even be said that a vaccine teaches or prompts the immune system to unleash its infection fighters against microbes that can harm us. It is prompted to do so by the vaccine.

By taking the special needs of older populations into account, scientists say it is possible to produce flu vaccines that help the aging immune system mount a more vigorous response. For vaccines to have optimal effectiveness two important components of the immune system must be part of the response: its recognition of a foreign invader and its ability to remember a previous one. Vaccines are composed of deactivated fragments of infectious microbes.

In a flu shot, a mere snippet of a deactivated virus is all that is used to help "teach" the immune system that the flu virus is a bad actor. Once the immune system "sees" the deactivated fragment, it then "remembers" it to produce antibodies. Antibodies, as explained in Question 55, are charged with remembering an influenza virus should it be encountered during flu season. Scientists, meanwhile, are taking that knowledge of vaccines and the immune system and applying it in their research for a seniors-only vaccine.

57. How does influenza cause people to die?

Influenza can act single handedly by causing viral pneumonia, or a flu infection can so weaken one's immune defenses that secondary bacterial invaders enter the lungs and become difficult to fight. Impairing the mechanism the body uses to clear inhaled bacteria from the lungs is one way in which a flu infection damages pulmonary function. Bacteria, especially microbes such as *Streptococcus pneumoniae* or *Staphylococcus aureus*, then can take advantage of the weakened condition and cause bacterial pneumonia. Studies have shown that when vaccination prevents influenza in the first place, the risk of secondary invaders is greatly diminished.

Streptococcus pneumoniae

A bacterial infection that can occur as a secondary condition in people debilitated by the flu.

Staphylococcus aureus

The most common cause of staph infections.

58. What is pneumonia?

Pneumonia is a disease as old as humankind itself and has been documented since the time of the ancients from cultures around the world. It is an extremely common respiratory infection and can occur among people of virtually any age, but deaths are most common among people who are very old, especially those whose immunity is compromised by other medical conditions. Pneumonia is an illness of the respiratory system in which the alveoli (air sacs) of the lungs become inflamed and filled with fluid, preventing the lungs from effectively utilizing oxygen. As just mentioned in Question 57, pneumonia has more than one cause: *S. pneumoniae* and *S. aureus* can lead to pneumonia, as can a number of other viruses, bacteria, and parasites. And although scientists have identified dozens of microbes that can cause pneumonia, only a few prove to be especially deadly. In addition to the flu virus, respiratory syncytial virus (RSV) can cause pneumonia; parainfluenza virus is another cause. Symptoms of pneumonia include labored breathing and fever.

59. Why are complications a concern in older people? What are some of the secondary illnesses that can occur as a result of influenza?

As mentioned earlier, the immune system's ability to respond efficiently wanes with age and our responses to infections become somewhat impaired. But this doesn't mean that influenza complications are primarily the domain of older adults. Secondary invaders—bacterial infections—do not discriminate based on age. Many people are susceptible to complications when the body has been weakened by influenza. Most of the complications that affect older people are the same ones that affect infants whose immune systems have yet to fully mature, as well as people in their teens and twenties who have underlying chronic conditions.

Secondary illnesses that can occur as a result of influenza are usually bacterial infections of the lower respiratory tract. One of the major bacterial invaders is pneumococcal pneumonia, triggered by the organism *S. pneumoniae*. It is a leading cause of serious illness in older adults—and children—worldwide. These bacteria are responsible for the majority of bacterial pneumonia cases in Western countries. In addition to pneumonia, *S. pneumoniae* can infiltrate the bloodstream, triggering a potentially lethal infection known as bacteremia. It also can invade the outer tissue lining of the brain to cause meningitis. The organism is a leading cause of strep throat, middle ear infections, and sinusitis. Serious infections can be treated effectively with antibiotics. Fortunately, an effective vaccine exists to prevent *S. pneumoniae* infections entirely.

60. What else should I know about pneumococcal pneumonia? Is there a vaccine?

The primary take-home message on **pneumococcal pneumonia** is that a protective vaccine exists for it—you don't have to get the infection. If your physician hasn't already recommended it, you may want to broach the subject yourself. The shot given to adults is technically called a polysaccharide vaccine, or PS 23. If you want to be vaccinated against pneumonia, you simply have to tell your doctor that you want the pneumonia shot.

pneumococcal pneumonia

A bacterial infection of the lungs which can occur alone or as a secondary infection in someone already affected by the flu.

Pneumonia vaccines have been available in the United States for more than three decades. In addition to reducing the risk of pneumonia, the vaccine also is associated with a reduced chance of respiratory failure, improved survival, and shorter hospital stays. The shot is designed to protect against the most common strains of *S. pneumoniae*. In all, scientists have identified more than 90 strains, but not all are associated with serious, invasive disease. Earlier versions of the vaccine protected against only 14 strains.

Healthcare providers can use one of two pneumococcal vaccines. Both are widely administered, and although many of the people who get the shots are 65 and older, the vaccines are not given exclusively to older people. Both are 23-valent vaccines, which means that they are aimed at providing protection against the 23 most common strains of *S. pneumoniae.*

One of the vaccines is known as Pneumovax, manufactured by Merck, Inc. Pneumovax was licensed by the U.S. Food and Drug Administration in 1977. Pnu-Imune 23, a product of Wyeth, was FDA approved in 1979.

Unlike the flu shot, which generally is administered in the fall, pneumococcal pneumonia vaccinations can be given at any time of the year. If you get the shot at the same time you are receiving a flu shot, your healthcare provider will administer it in the opposite arm.

Guarding against pneumococcal pneumonia is important because the infection is a serious source of illness and death. The National Network for Immunization Information estimates that more than 40,000 people in the United States are infected annually and about 4,425 die as a direct result of invasive pneumococcal disease. Government health officials further estimate that more than half of all cases and nearly all of the deaths occurred among adults who could have avoided infection had they been vaccinated.

61. Does Medicare pay for flu and pneumococcal vaccinations?

Medicare Part B assumes the cost of both the flu and pneumococcal pneumonia shots.

62. Can broader vaccination programs for children aid older people?

Public health authorities answer with an emphatic yes, but they add a few caveats. Even though the purpose of vaccinating youngsters against the flu is first and foremost aimed at protecting each child, there is strong evidence demonstrating that when more children are immunized, there are added benefits for society as a whole. According to the Childhood Influenza Coalition, which is part of the National Foundation for Infectious Diseases, "widespread childhood flu vaccination can interrupt influenza transmission because outbreaks usually begin among children and then move to the community at large."

Blocking widespread flu transmission within the age group most likely to spread the infection bolsters herd immunity, the kind of immunity that occurs when immunization levels are so high in the greater population (the herd) that even unvaccinated people are protected. With respect to influenza, children are key constituents of the herd. When the CDC's advisory committee recommended in February 2008 that children between the ages of 6 months and 18 years receive an annual flu vaccination, the panel noted that reducing flu transmission among children has the added benefit of reducing influenza prevalence throughout communities.

Older people should not avoid vaccination simply because there are more immunization programs for youngsters. Individual protection among older people, experts say, is what counts most in guarding against influenza. Regardless of age, vaccination is the most effective way to avoid secondary illnesses and hospitalization that are associated with the flu.

PART SIX

Outbreaks, Epidemics, and Pandemics

What are some important points to know about epidemics?

Why do flu viruses spread in winter?
Does weather affect the way influenza is transmitted?

Clearly, some pandemics are worse than others.
Do health agencies have a way of knowing in advance
how bad a pandemic will be?

More . . .

63. What are some important points to know about epidemics?

The most obvious reason influenza is to be considered with utmost seriousness is based on its potential to spread quickly through communities. Infections are tracked by municipal, state, national, and global public health agencies because of the flu's potential to spawn outbreaks, which, in turn, can develop into wider clusters of infection in a relatively short period of time. Flu outbreaks not only have the potential to spread, they carry the threat of secondary illnesses that can adversely affect vulnerable segments of the population.

outbreak

A sudden rise in the incidence of a disease.

An **outbreak** in an elementary or middle school, for instance, suggests the potential for each child to carry the infection home and thus promote influenza's spread in the larger community. Dr. Michael Greger, director of Public Health and Animal Agriculture at the Humane Society of the United States, notes that infections in school-age children can mean death for grandparents at home. Infant siblings are also at elevated risk of death.

In a full-blown flu epidemic, the hale and hardy are usually feverish and miss work or school for a few days. But epidemiologists have long underscored that the key hallmarks of a flu epidemic are a sharp increase in hospital admissions for pneumonia and a rise in the number of deaths from that respiratory condition. Inevitably, the brunt of flu-related risks hit hardest among those least able to mount an effective immune response: babies, the elderly, and people with respiratory and immune-compromising medical conditions. Despite centuries of coping with flu, widespread influenza epidemics remain unavoidable.

Dr. Pascal James Imperato, a former health commissioner for New York City, wrote in his book *What to Do About the Flu* that "many of the so-called plagues of ancient times were actually flu epidemics. But they [were] so poorly described that medical historians cannot properly include them in the history of the flu." The Bible is full of references to sweeping plagues that have all the hallmarks of flu epidemics.

The term *epidemic*, Dr. Imperato emphasizes, simply means that many people in a given locale become sick within a relatively short period of time. Health agencies, such as the Centers for Disease Control and Prevention and the World Health Organization, use sophisticated mathematical measurements to decide whether an epidemic is under way. For example, epidemiologists examine the rate at which a disease occurs during a specific period, calculating the number of new cases against what is expected based on previous experience. The number of new cases compared with the number of expected cases is called the incidence rate. A substantial spike in the incidence rate can lead health authorities to declare an epidemic.

The term *epidemic* has taken on broader meaning over the years to include conditions that are noninfectious. You very likely may have heard of the obesity epidemic, the suicide epidemic, and even the homeless epidemic. In those instances, epidemiologists also are measuring the number of cases that would be expected compared with those they've actually calculated.

Seasonal flu epidemics are noteworthy because of the many ways in which the infection moves through a population. Sometimes an epidemic has a slow start, beginning with only a few incidents before exploding into scores of cases. In other instances, the onset is explosive, and then trickles to only a few. Transmission dynamics are innumerable and illustrative of the ways in which flu viruses are being transmitted from one person to the next.

An additional point about flu epidemics cannot be stressed more emphatically: Public health agencies—local and global—track influenza activity because of the ease with which the infection is passed person to person. Even though there is some blurring of lines when it comes to differentiating an outbreak from an epidemic, there is a very definite distinction between an epidemic and a pandemic.

A flu pandemic is not an epidemic that has grown larger, spreading around the world. An influenza pandemic refers to rare, globe-circling waves of illness caused by a flu strain that is new to human populations. No one—young, old, or those in between—has any form of antibody protection. There were only three flu pandemics during the 20th century. By comparison there were so many outbreaks and epidemics that it is likely no healthcare agency has an accurate count.

64. How do health authorities know when an epidemic is under way?

Health authorities have a variety of ways of assessing flu activity in communities, even though they never get an accurate head count because most people self-treat influenza and never see a physician. When hospitalizations for the flu and pneumonia exceed seasonal thresholds and people are dying of respiratory infections in higher than expected numbers, public health authorities know that the makings of an epidemic are probably under way.

Declarations of epidemics in the United States are based on several factors, including an assessment of laboratory-confirmed cases of influenza. State health departments study laboratory specimens from patients, isolating and identifying the type of flu virus that has caused infection. Doing so gives health officials a sense of which strain or strains are being transmitted most frequently.

Local and state health departments often gather data during flu season from a network of medical personnel who provide flu-related information based on cases they are treating. In many states throughout the United States, emergency room doctors, hospital laboratories, and sentinel physicians—private practice doctors whose offices fill with coughing, achy patients during flu season—report laboratory-confirmed cases to local and state health departments. As part of this reporting, cases of pneumonia and pneumonia-related deaths are also conveyed to local and state health authorities.

 Among the combination of signals alerting state health authorities to a flu epidemic are an excess number of laboratory-confirmed flu cases and an excess number of pneumonia deaths, especially deaths occurring among children. Each state has thresholds that aid in determining how many flu cases and pneumonia deaths are considered excessive.

State epidemiologists, who monitor flu activity, maintain running tallies of laboratory-confirmed cases. Most U.S. state health departments post weekly maps on their Web sites providing details for the public. The maps are colored to mark areas of flu activity and indicate whether it is low, moderate, or high. All states routinely report flu activity data to the Centers for Disease Control and Prevention, which conducts national influenza surveillance. As part of its monitoring, the CDC maintains a tally of pneumonia cases treated at 122 selected hospitals during flu season. The hospitals provide a representative cross-section of flu-related pneumonia in the United States. Data from the hospital network can help CDC epidemiologists determine when a flu epidemic is under way nationwide.

65. If a flu pandemic is not an epidemic that gets out of hand, what causes it?

Pandemics occur when a unique influenza A virus abruptly enters human populations, spawned through a process called antigenic shift. Shifted viruses possess a radically new arrangement of coat proteins—hemagglutinin and neuraminidase—that stipple the viral surface. Flu viruses use those proteins to commandeer human cells. Antigenic shift produces a pandemic strain, a virus that not only is deadly but can spread around the world with frightening speed. A shifted virus can emerge in human populations in one of three ways (see **Figure 3**):

1. A bird flu strain might jump directly from aquatic fowl to humans where it can undergo further genetic change and become easily transmitted person to person.
2. An aquatic bird through its feces or urine can pass viruses to an intermediary host, such as a chicken or pig.
3. A new strain can spread from a chicken or pig to humans.

When a shifted virus develops the genetic characteristics allowing simple person-to-person transmission (as with seasonal flu), the strain has acquired the necessary properties to fuel a pandemic. Pandemic flu is animal-to-human infection followed by mutations that aid simple person-to-person transmission of a strain to which humans have no natural immunity.

Theoretically, an animal virus can become easily transmissible if it jumps to a person who also happens to be infected with a seasonal flu strain. In that instance the animal and human flu strains might intermingle, causing the genetic material from the two viruses to undergo reassortment. **Reassortment**, a mixing of genes, conceivably can produce a novel pathogen capable of emerging as a pandemic strain.

reassortment

A rearrangements of genes that emanates from two distinct strains of influenza.

This intermingling of genes is often called the "mixing bowl" effect, and there is more than one way in which it can occur. Pigs are well known as a species that can become infected with human flu viruses as well as those from birds. Human and avian flu pathogens can intermingle in the pig, exchanging genes. It is possible that the emergent virus could spread from the intermediary to humans as a pandemic strain.

U.S. federal health officials in 1976 feared pigs would be the source of a monstrous global outbreak, acting as mixing bowls for a pandemic flu. Their theories, of course, didn't pan out.

The take-home message here is simple: Antigenic shift can produce a radically new A subtype virus. When this happens, the age-old patterns of coughing, sneezing, shaking hands, or touching contaminated objects can quickly transmit a devastatingly lethal infection around the world. Each of the three pandemics that struck during the 20th century was caused by a unique strain that occurred through antigenic shift.

66. Why are epidemics different? Is antigenic shift involved?

Unlike pandemics, which are caused only by novel influenza A subtypes, epidemics can be caused by either seasonal A or B viruses. These pathogens are not nearly as threatening as pandemic strains, and have no connection to the process of antigenic shift. Seasonal flu viruses are, however, in constant flux—changing in infinitesimal ways. The tiny changes made by seasonal flu viruses are known as antigenic drift. The flu viruses we encounter each year have undergone—and are undergoing—some degree of drift. Knowing that drift occurs can help you understand a critical influenza conundrum, basically why people are never fully immune to it.

We can catch the flu more than once because antigenic drift causes flu viruses to change their H and N identity ever so slightly. The change is just enough to keep the human immune system a bit uncertain—questioning—whether this was the culprit it had seen the previous year, or whether it was another. Ongoing, subtle changes help explain why influenza viruses remain continuously infectious.

A couple of other important points about antigenic drift and shift can help put these concepts into better perspective. Antigenic shift is a major, unusual change that can lead to a pandemic flu strain. Pandemics are rare. Antigenic drift refers to small, constant changes that can underlie an epidemic in some flu seasons or mild influenza activity in others. Antigenic drift never creates the seismic change associated with antigenic shift.

67. If epidemics are not rare, how frequently do they occur? Are some epidemics worse than others?

As mind-boggling as it may seem, epidemics occur almost every flu season, somewhere in the world. In the United States, federal health officials have documented serious flu epidemics every 2 to 3 years. Nothing about this cycling is cast in stone (see Question 63). The reasons for flu epidemics abound.

Flu viruses may get a jump on the season, flaring earlier than expected and causing waves of infections before sufficient numbers of people have been vaccinated. Outbreaks in schools may lead to wider-than-expected cases in communities. Sometimes the vaccine may not be ideal. On occasion, as was the case during the 2007–2008 influenza season, there may be a mismatch between a circulating strain of the flu and the one in the vaccine. Lower levels of protection in communities as a whole lead to a higher incidence of infection.

Yet, even though epidemics occur frequently, that does not mean waves of infection are spreading throughout an entire country, especially one the size of the United States. Federal epidemiologists have often noted that flu activity may be high in some regions of the country and virtually inactive elsewhere. The difference depends on a variety of factors, including how many people in a given population have been vaccinated and therefore have been guarded against infection.

There are still other reasons for flu epidemics, many of which can lead to devastating outcomes particularly in resource-poor nations where vaccination levels are low to nonexistent.

Poverty and malnutrition can make a bout with the flu deadly. In 2002, a flu epidemic swept across Madagascar, killing 650 people and infecting 22,000, according to data from the World Health Organization. The deadly epidemic was caused by an H3N2 strain, a seasonal virus that initially seemed to possess pandemic strength. Massive waves of illness disabled thousands. WHO doctors, dispatched to the island nation off the coast of Africa, blamed the epidemic's rapid spread on impoverished living conditions, malnutrition, and the inability of the people to secure effective medical treatment.

When Madagascans developed pneumonia as a consequence of the flu, they could not afford antibiotics to treat the secondary infections. Already weakened by inadequate food intake and poor hydration, many who were stricken simply lacked the physical strength to effectively fight the infection. Flu epidemics, such as the one in Madagascar, can become explosive forces.

68. Are epidemics caused by A strains more virulent than those caused by influenza B viruses?

When you are infected with an A or B influenza virus you will not know which one made you sick. Both make you feel miserable. But there is a subtle difference between the epidemics spawned by the two viral types. (You may recall from earlier in the discussion that there are three types of influenza viruses: A, B, and C. Type C flu viruses are not associated with epidemics.)

Type A viruses are notorious for their link to epidemics and have been associated with noteworthy epidemics worldwide. Epidemiologists estimate that in the United States seasonal A viruses are responsible for epidemics roughly every 2 to 3 years. Influenza B viruses have been associated with epidemics approximately every 3 to 5 years. There is yet another distinction between epidemics caused by A and B influenza viruses:

B viruses tend to cause less-severe epidemics. However, these viruses, which exclusively infect humans, are still associated with pneumonia and death.

Seasonal flu epidemics, whether caused by A or B viruses, tend to occur in two waves. The first usually is associated with school-age children and members of their households; the second wave generally is detected among institutionalized patients, most notably elderly people in nursing homes.

69. Why do flu viruses spread in winter? Does weather affect the way influenza is transmitted?

One of the enduring anecdotes about the flu is that epidemics seem to be worse when the weather dips to its coldest temperatures. On a basic level, that is easy to understand. People are more likely to be indoors and in closer contact when the weather is chilly outdoors. Schools plan more indoor activities for students when it's cold, especially in places where it snows—again, providing more opportunities for close contact and the transmission of influenza. But some people believe that it's actually the cold—the frigidness of the weather—that aids in the flu's transmission.

For generations, mothers worldwide have encouraged children to bundle up as protection against the flu, another sign that people have long associated cold weather with catching influenza. Now, scientific analysis is lending credence to the anecdotes, even suggesting that mothers may have been right, albeit only partially so. Yes, cold, dry weather does play a role in viral transmission, but putting on a warm coat doesn't prevent you from getting the flu.

In a groundbreaking series of experiments in which guinea pigs "caught" the flu, a team of medical investigators at Mount Sinai Medical School in New York City confirmed that cooler temperatures and dry air conspire to help influenza spread more efficiently. The researchers found that flu viruses simply persist longer when the temperature is lower and the air dry. And as other scientists not connected with this research have demonstrated, mucus is thicker during winter months, providing a welcome environment for the pathogen to persist in nasal passages. Hence, with coughing, sneezing, or even talking to someone at close range, the virus is more likely to be transmitted from one person to the next, especially when conditions for its persistence are ideal. The guinea pig study, which was reported in 2007 in the online journal *PloS* (Public Library of Science), provides yet additional evidence that cold, dry weather could very well be a factor in how effectively influenza spreads.

The Mount Sinai team didn't arrive at its conclusion easily—and they didn't start their study with a ready supply of guinea pigs, animals that have not been routinely used in scientific research for decades. As part of the research, Dr. Peter Palese, lead investigator of the analysis, turned to information from the great pandemic of 1918 for answers.

Palese found a scientific investigation from the era that was particularly tantalizing. U.S. Army doctors at Camp Cody in New Mexico reported extensively in a 1919 edition of the *Journal of the American Medical Association* that the lethal pandemic not only ravaged their troops, it also killed their laboratory guinea pigs. In the early 20th century, guinea pigs were widely used in scientific research. The *JAMA* report, nevertheless, leapt out at Palese for an important reason: It revealed an animal model that could catch the same influenza that infects humans.

The team began their experiments by exposing some of the guinea pigs to a flu strain that normally affects humans. Guinea pigs caught the flu when scientists inoculated the animals' nasal passages. The wide-eyed rodents with prominent ears were housed in small chambers that allowed air to flow from infected animals to those that were healthy.

Even though guinea pigs do not cough or sneeze, they do, like any other mammal, exhale. Sick guinea pigs, the scientists discovered, passed the infection to healthy animals simply through the air they exhaled. This became most evident when scientists adjusted the temperature and humidity in the chambers, essentially simulating various weather conditions.

Flu transmission, the team discovered, was inversely correlated with temperature and relative humidity. In other words, the lower the temperature and the lower the relative humidity, the more likely that flu-stricken guinea pigs would transmit their infection. Flu transmission was most efficient at 5° Celsius (41° Fahrenheit) and low relative humidity.

Even at room temperature, flu transmission peaked at low relative humidity (low relative humidity is in the range of 20% to 35%). By comparison, flu transmission decreased when relative humidity reached 50%. At 80% humidity, transmission dropped off. So, the cooler and drier the air, the easier it was for the flu to be passed from sick animals to their healthy counterparts. The group of collaborators conducted a series of 20 experiments to reach this conclusion.

Scientists who critiqued the research said the discovery furthers the understanding of influenza transmission and highlights how cooler, drier weather can aid the spread of flu viruses between individuals, and possibly even among ever-increasing numbers of people as influenza spreads in an epidemic.

70. What were the major flu pandemics of the 20th century?

There were three major globe-girdling pandemics that killed millions of people in the last century. Each of these outbreaks still provides valuable lessons for epidemiologists who are studying the potential for a global pandemic today:

- 1918—Sometimes called the Spanish flu or the mother of all pandemics, this outbreak killed more people in 12 weeks than those who died in World War I. And even though the pandemic is often called the Spanish flu, it didn't begin in Spain. The term has been misleading for nearly a century. The infections were spawned by H1N1, a virus identified decades after the pandemic. Virologists today say H1N1 was uniquely lethal. An estimated 50 million people died, but the death toll may have been as high as 100 million. Medical scientists in 1918 had no idea what type of pathogen caused the devastating waves of illness, although they were well aware of the infection's extreme contagiousness. Public health officials ordered a number of nonpharmaceutical precautions to prevent the spread of influenza, such as requiring people to wear masks and closing theaters and other places where people gather in large numbers. Some communities were better at implementing these measures than others and as a result were able to spare more lives.
- 1957—The Asian flu was caused by pandemic strain H2N2. An estimated two million people died worldwide. Global health authorities suspected a pandemic was developing when 250,000 cases of influenza quickly swept through Hong Kong. Scientists in the United States, Great Britain, and Australia collaborated in a major scientific effort to isolate and identify the virus, which they found to be one that had undergone antigenic shift, a signal that they were dealing with a pandemic strain.
- 1968—The Hong Kong flu is another pandemic with a name that does not quite reflect its origin. This flu virus is believed to have originated in Southeast Asia and was caused by H3N2. An estimated one million people died worldwide. Descendants of this virus now circulate as seasonal flu viruses.

71. Clearly, some pandemics are worse than others. Do health agencies have a way of knowing in advance how bad a pandemic will be?

The U.S. Department of Health and Human Services and the Centers for Disease Control and Prevention in 2007 developed a measure called the Pandemic Severity Index, or PSI. It is very similar to the approach involved in describing hurricanes, and likewise consists of five categories. A category 1 pandemic is comparable to a severe seasonal epidemic. The difference between the two is the type of virus causing the infections. A severe seasonal epidemic is triggered by a seasonal flu virus; a category 1 pandemic is caused by a shifted virus that is new to human populations. On the other end of the scale, a category 5 pandemic is one with devastating consequences, such as the 1918 flu—or worse.

Health authorities declare a category 1, 2, 3, 4, or 5 pandemic based on the flu's death rate. When the percentage of infected people is high and accompanied by a high death rate, the PSI is correspondingly high, warranting a designation of category 4 or 5. When the percentage of infected people is moderate and the death rate is relatively low, the PSI is low. The 1968 Hong Kong flu is considered a category 1 pandemic. The 1957 flu pandemic is considered a category 2.

72. Wasn't there a scare involving the resurgence of the 1957 pandemic flu strain?

The 1957 flu strain did not reemerge, but a frightening mishap occurred between September 2004 and March 2005 that created a stir in the scientific community. Vials of the 1957 pandemic strain were accidentally shipped to laboratories worldwide. News media "talking heads" speculated about the possibility of reigniting the 1957 pandemic, but a resurgence of the strain never became an issue. The error was caught and global health authorities intervened, ordering the vials to be destroyed. The incident reinvigorated the very real—and ongoing—concern of proper labeling and control of dangerous pathogens.

The vials were shipped to laboratories in a kit as part of required accreditation testing. Meridian Bioscience, Inc., in Cincinnati, which dispatched the kits by overnight mail to nearly 4,000 laboratories worldwide, prepared the laboratory testing materials for the College of American Pathologists. The college accredits laboratories and requires that labs seeking its certification demonstrate an ability to identify specific pathogens, including an A strain of flu. Many of the labs receiving a vial of the 1957 pandemic strain were located in hospitals. Alert scientists in Canada recognized the virus as the killer pandemic strain that circumnavigated the globe in the 1950s and quickly notified the World Health Organization.

Meridian officials chose the 1957 virus because it was classified for use in a biosafety level-2 (BSL-2) lab. Laboratories with this designation routinely handle influenza viruses, as well as other infectious viruses and bacteria. When the mishap was discovered, scientists overwhelmingly agreed that the 1957 flu strain should be handled only by BSL-3 laboratories, a type of laboratory with much tighter security measures.

In all, there are four biosafety levels: BSL-1, BSL-2, BSL-3, and BSL-4. Containment measures increase according to the designation of the lab. Measures are not as stringent in a BSL-1 lab as they are in a BSL-2 lab; containment measures in a BSL-2 lab are not as stringent as they are in a BSL-3 lab, and so on.

What wasn't widely known at the time the kits were shipped was that the 1957 strain could have proven lethal to anyone born after 1957. People born after this year now make up the majority of the world's population. And because this segment of the world's population was never exposed to the virus, millions lacked even a trace of immunity against it. The company had no idea that it was shipping a potentially lethal strain.

Both the WHO and the Centers for Disease Control and Prevention issued terse warnings as soon as it was discovered that the virus had been accidentally shipped. The two health agencies demanded the vials' destruction.

Known as H2N2, the strain was first reported in northern China in the early months of 1956. But it was not until the following year that it sparked the 1957 Asian flu pandemic that quickly spread around the world. Among the estimated two million people who died in that deadly flu season were 69,000 who perished in the United States. Dr. Gary Leonardi, a virologist at Nassau University Medical Center in New York, was among those who mistakenly received the flu strain. He said the sample arrived in a lyophilized state (freeze-dried), which means it had to be reconstituted with water to become infectious. The sample weighed 2 milligrams, he said, which in a reconstituted state would have been equivalent to about 40 drops of fluid from an eyedropper.

At the time the kits were shipped, the CDC was drafting documents to reclassify the 1957 pandemic strain as a BSL-3 pathogen. It was estimated that many laboratories, such as Meridian, probably had the 1957 pandemic strain in their viral libraries and were unaware of its lethal potential. BSL-3 laboratories have specific design features in which strict attention is paid to airflow. Laboratory scientists and technicians must conduct their work under special containment devices and wear protective eyewear and clothing. Pathogens handled in BSL-3 labs are exceptionally threatening. They include *Bacillus anthrasis*, which causes anthrax, the severe acute respiratory syndrome (SARS) virus, and the tuberculosis bacillus, to name a few.

73. Do pandemics follow the same wintertime prevalence pattern seen with seasonal flu?

A characteristic of pandemic flu viruses is their unpredictability. They do not follow the "rules" established by their seasonal influenza counterparts. Dr. Jeffrey Taubenberger, one of the world's leading 1918 flu experts, wrote in the journal *Emerging Infectious Diseases* that historical records dating back to the 16th century suggest pandemics can appear at any time of year. Globe-sweeping pandemics, Taubenberger theorizes, do not surface in the usual late-year pattern consistent with seasonal influenza. Pandemic strains tend to smolder, sometimes for months, if not years, as research now suggests was the case prior to each of the global outbreaks of the last century. The smoldering effect is one reason why disease detectives from the World Health Organization are monitoring the avian virus H5N1 as birds continue to spread it around the world. Flu experts want to make certain that among people who contract it, the virus does not undergo the genetic changes allowing it to become easily transmissible. Should that happen, the world then might face an emergent pandemic strain, one that could first smolder in a hot zone of infection before taking off in a global wave of influenza.

Newly "shifted" viruses, according to Taubenberger, "behave differently when they find a universal or highly susceptible human population." A former chief of molecular pathology at the Armed Forces Institute of Pathology in Washington, D.C., Taubenberger theorizes that illnesses linked to the 1918 pandemic strain probably started years before the worst waves of influenza struck in the fall and winter of 1918–1919. This is what is meant by a smoldering effect.

Unlike seasonal influenza, which arrives annually like clockwork, the pandemic probably got a sputtering start before picking up gale force strength as it sped around the world. The complex outbreak is still raising questions about transmission dynamics, the number of affected countries, and how a pandemic differs from a seasonal flu epidemic. The report in *Emerging Infectious Diseases* underscores that an elevated number of respiratory illnesses were first noted in the United States as early as 1915. The infections continued through

1916, dipped somewhat in 1917 before emerging in a wave of devastating illnesses in the spring of 1918. The explosive waves that followed in the fall and winter are the ones for which the pandemic became notorious. An estimated 50 million people died in a matter of only a few months, although some estimates put the global death toll as high as 100 million.

Spurred by an H1N1 viral strain, which had never before infected humans, it is very likely the pandemic virus had been around for years. Peering through a modern lens, researchers now say there was a simultaneous flu outbreak in U.S. swine in 1918 that might have added clues and context to the pandemic that gripped the world's human populations—if scientists of the day knew what to look for. But the medical community in 1918 possessed very limited tools to understand what was in their midst.

Modern scientists who have reconstructed the deadly 1918 virus and studied it in the laboratory say they have gleaned a very simple message from history: Pandemic viruses do not abide by the rules nature established for seasonal strains. And because pandemic viruses do not play by the usual rules, researchers are still learning new lessons about a pandemic that occurred nearly 100 years ago. Contemporary experts say the virus did not crop up overnight and that it may have taken years to evolve into a global killer.

Taubenberger asks this question: "Is it possible that a poorly adapted H1N1 was already beginning to spread in 1915, causing some serious illnesses but not yet sufficiently fit to initiate a pandemic?" Taubenberger's theory, which suggests the pandemic got its start years before the explosive 1918 event, is consistent with observations in Europe reported by British military doctors in 1916. Contemporary analyses by a British virologist also suggest the first illnesses probably began years before 1918. Taken together, the modern American and British retrospective studies compellingly underscore that pandemics do not begin abruptly in a specific season but smolder insidiously before exploding in waves of infections that race around the world.

PART SEVEN

Keeping the 1918 Pandemic in Mind

Why is the 1918 flu pandemic so important?

If the flu virus wasn't identified until the 1930s, how did public health officials in 1918 know what they were dealing with?

Are there any practical lessons to be learned from the 1918 pandemic?

More . . .

74. Why is the 1918 flu pandemic so important?

The 1918 pandemic was triggered by an extraordinarily contagious form of influenza that rapidly sped around the globe through what now seems unbelievably simple chains of close human contact: coughing, sneezing, shaking hands, kissing, perhaps even holding conversations at close range. Everyone at the time had a brush with the illness in an exceptionally personal way. Either they were infected with the flu and came within a whisper of death, or they knew someone who contracted it. Virtually everyone knew someone who died.

Nothing quite like the magnitude of this global plague has occurred since, not even the two other flu pandemics that struck later in the 20th century. Experts now agree the 1918 flu virus—H1N1—was unique, but that doesn't mean the pandemic was so unique that nothing like it will ever occur again. Another pandemic of that strength—or worse—can emerge, according to experts who study pandemics and influenza. That is why global surveillance of flu viruses remains one of the core activities of the World Health Organization, the CDC, and other agencies of disease detectives.

Critical public health questions about the 1918 pandemic persist despite the fact that the waves of illness occurred at the beginning of the last century. Studies of death certificates from the era reveal the pandemic produced a W-shaped mortality rate rather than the U-shaped curve that might have been expected. What does this mean? Rather than the elevated number of deaths among babies, very low mortality among adults, and elevated death rate in the elderly—which, when plotted, forms the traditional U-shaped curve—analyses reveal a completely different story. Yes, there was high mortality among babies and toddlers, but the death rate dipped among older children, and then sharply rose for young adults between the ages of 20 and 40, and there was another sharp rise in deaths among the frail elderly to complete the **W-shaped curve**. Discovering who was most vulnerable in the

W-curve

A curve that reflects the pattern of deaths from the 1918 pandemic. There were a large number of deaths among infants, people aged 18-40, and the elderly.

pandemic and who was able to escape it came as a surprise to contemporary investigators who were startled by the mortality peak for people between the ages of 20 and 40, usually among any society's healthiest.

During the first annual conference on Seasonal and Pandemic Flu in Arlington, Virginia, in 2007, one presenter included as part of her report dozens of pictures that illustrated the meaning of the W-shaped curve. Photo after photo of gravestones revealed birth and death dates of young men and women in their early 20s, mid-20s, and early 30s. Some had been soldiers and sailors in World War I (see **Figure 6**). Others were young husbands and wives, some only in their late teens, buried together with their infants, all victims of pandemic influenza.

Studies of medical records from the era also revealed other surprises. Although children between the ages of 5 and 14

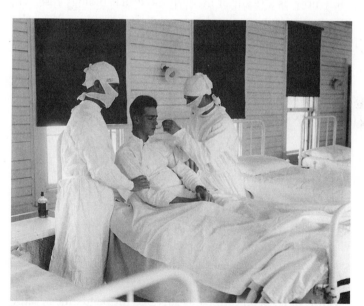

Figure 6   Two nurses treating an influenza patient at Naval Hospital New Orleans, Louisiana, circa 1918.
Courtesy of Naval Historical Center.

accounted for a disproportionate number of flu cases, they also had a much lower death rate from influenza and pneumonia than other age groups. There also was a lower-than-expected death rate for middle-aged adults. Healthy elderly people, surprisingly, tended to survive the pandemic. Contemporary flu hunters say the 1918 pandemic remains mystifying and enduringly instructive.

"Today, nearly a century after the 1918 influenza pandemic, its mysteries remain largely unexplained," Dr. Anthony Fauci, director of the National Institute of Allergy and Infectious Diseases, said in a 2007 statement. "Much work remains to be done, by scientists as well as by historians and other scholars, with regard to the many unanswered questions surrounding this historic pandemic. These studies must be part of our preparedness efforts as we face the prospect of a future influenza pandemic."

Only now, as a result of modern molecular biology research, have scientists begun to develop a clearer picture of why the young and robust—in the prime of health and strength—were among the pandemic's primary victims. A possible explanation, which has been reinforced through studies of mice involving a reconstructed version of the 1918 virus, is that young people probably died of an overactive immune response.

cytokine storm

A potentially lethal immune system response to infection, marked by an abrupt surge in pro-inflammatory proteins known as cytokines.

Dr. Fauci and other scientists suggest young adults succumbed to a **cytokine storm**, which is described as an excessive flood of immune system proteins that spur an overwhelming inflammatory response. The powerful immune system of young adults betrays the body in its open assault on the invading virus. Like turncoats, the warrior constituents of the immune system do more damage than the infection itself.

Healthy older people probably survived the pandemic because their immune systems were not as aggressive and did not fight the viral invasion with such force—at least that is the most potent theory. Many grandparents, great aunts, and great uncles suddenly found themselves rearing children, scores of whom were orphaned by the plague. For many young adults, youth offered no reprieve from the inevitable. At the height of the pandemic, the time from onset of initial symptoms to death was often swift.

A contemporary comparison can be made with the deaths of people infected with H5N1, the bird flu virus. Most who have succumbed to the virus have been under the age of 40. However, experts have yet to determine whether a higher percentage of young people die compared with older people and whether younger people are more susceptible to infection and death because they are more likely to be exposed to birds.

75. Why is the 1918 pandemic associated with Spain?

The term Spanish flu, which has been widely used to designate the outbreak of 1918, is a misnomer. Contemporary analyses of medical reports from the era have brought new insight into the beginnings of the infections that eventually became a global pandemic. No one knows precisely where the pandemic began—or when—but scientists now have several strong theories. They're absolutely certain that the global pandemic of 1918 did not emerge in Spain. Spain, unlike other countries with a growing number of sick people, did not censor the fact that thousands were becoming ill. The country was, however, the first to acknowledge publicly that something contagious—but initially nonfatal—was spreading through the population. Spain probably got stuck with "Spanish flu" because of its openness about its population being stricken with a strange new disease.

The news media of that time can also be blamed for spreading the term Spanish flu. During the spring of 1918, the Spanish news organization *Agencia Fabra* sent a cable to London, reporting an unusual respiratory illness. The report, which was sent to the Reuters news service, noted that people throughout Madrid were falling ill. At that time, in late spring, during the first wave of illnesses, deaths apparently had not yet escalated because the report stressed common symptoms, such as cough, fever, headache, and the illness running its course in a few days. As the alerts from Spain continued, the news worsened and the country ultimately documented eight million cases of influenza. Perhaps because of Spain's ongoing reports about an ever-expanding outbreak it became indelibly linked to the flu.

76. You've referred to waves of illness in the 1918 pandemic. How many waves were there?

Most contemporary theorists estimate a series of waves characterized the 1918 global flu pandemic. The first wave occurred in the spring of 1918, the second in the fall of that year, and in some countries but not all, a third wave ignited illnesses in the early part of 1919. The initial spring wave arose at a time of year that is not favorable to influenza's spread. The calamitous second wave, however, caused simultaneous outbreaks in the Northern and Southern Hemispheres, sweeping violently through populations from September to November. An equally violent third wave continued through the early months of 1919. By the end of spring in 1919, the pandemic had run its course.

77. How many people were infected?

Disease detectives who now study the 1918 pandemic estimate that one-third of the world's population was infected during any one of the three major waves of illness that girdled the globe at the end of World War I. In terms of raw numbers, 500 million people were infected. The number of deaths, which typically is estimated between 40 to 50 million, may have been dramatically higher. The true number will never be known because many countries did not maintain vital statistics. What is known with absolute certainty is that the majority of deaths occurred within only 12 weeks. Nothing so extraordinarily devastating has occurred since then.

Every continent with the exception of Antarctica was affected by the pandemic. Along the icy Seward Peninsula in Alaska, home to the Inuit people, the pandemic nearly wiped out the tiny igloo-dwelling community. More than 70 adults died in the pandemic, leaving 46 children behind. In other less-developed parts of the world, there is evidence that the flu struck, but no one has any idea how many people died.

In the United States, 28% of the population was infected and between 500,000 and 675,000 people perished. In some hard-hit cities, such as Philadelphia, so many people died there were not enough gravediggers to bury the dead. An estimated 400,000 died in France, 250,000 in Great Britain, and 50,000 in Canada. India lost nearly 3% of its population. An estimated 7 million people throughout the country died in the pandemic. Populations in Africa and remote Pacific islands were decimated. So many people were killed by the flu in Africa that contemporary epidemiologists say it would be impossible to estimate the tens of millions of people who died. Millions of children around the world were orphaned.

Some made light of a dark time in their lives. A childhood rhyme from the era is a reminder of what seemed to be a threat lurking at every open window:

> *I had a little bird its name was Enza*
> *I opened the window, and*
> *In-Flew-Enza*

Some adults who experienced the horror posited theories of German biological warfare. Pulitzer Prize–winning author Katherine Anne Porter, who was a 28-year-old newspaper reporter in 1918 working at the *Rocky Mountain News* in

Denver, nearly died in the pandemic. She advanced the notion of influenza as a possible biological weapon in the semiautobiographical 1939 trilogy *Pale Horse, Pale Rider*: "They say that it is really caused by germs brought by a German ship to Boston," one of Porter's characters states flatly. "Somebody reported seeing a strange, thick, greasy-looking cloud float up out of Boston Harbor."

Scientists now know the viral culprit was a new pathogen with an unprecedented ability to generate waves of lethal illness that rapidly circled the globe.

78. If the flu virus wasn't identified until the 1930s, how did public health officials in 1918 know what they were dealing with?

Public health officials did not know specifically what had hit virtually every city, town, village, and remote outpost all over the world. They did know the infection had all of the hallmarks of the seasonal affliction they called influenza, which is why it was diagnosed as such—influenza was not a new disease. Doctors in 1918 were stymied because they could not pinpoint the causative agent. Since the 19th century, physicians believed influenza was triggered by a bacterium, *Hemophilus influenzae*. Indeed, the bacterium was named influenzae because the scientist who discovered it was convinced the microbe caused the flu.

German physician and bacteriologist Friedrich Johann Pfeiffer identified the bacterium and named it after isolating the pathogen from specimens of people stricken in the 1889–1890 flu epidemic. The organism was also known as Pfeiffer's bacillus.

But physicians and scientists in 1918 who studied specimens from pandemic victims were puzzled when they found *H. influenzae* in only a few samples but not in a majority. If *H. influenzae* was, in fact, the cause, why wasn't it turning up in all of their specimens? Ultimately, in the early 1930s, Dr. Richard Shope isolated a virus as the cause of influenza. He first found that the pathogen caused influenza in swine, and shortly afterward discovered that a virus was the cause of influenza in humans.

As for *H. influenzae*, medical scientists now recognize it as a secondary infection that can sometimes affect those suffering from the flu. This type of bacterial invasion is also more formally called an opportunistic infection. Scientists have identified six subtypes, the most notable of which is *H. influenzae* type B, which can cause serious childhood infections and now is sometimes called "daycare disease." Most doctors simply refer to it as Hib. Vaccines exist to prevent it.

79. Without significant air travel how was the virus spread to so many countries?

Troops were being moved all over Europe and throughout the United States. Barracks and ships at home and abroad were crowded with soldiers and sailors who could easily pass the infection to each other. Sick military personnel who returned to their hometowns also brought with them a deadly souvenir picked up during stints overseas. But the spread of influenza went beyond the military. Products were being shipped all over the world through vast trade networks that involved countries rich and poor, industrialized, feudal, and even tribal. Trade routes are believed to be the deadly pathways that brought the flu to the Eskimos who inhabited the icy permafrost region of Alaska. Populations were affected in distant Pacific islands and throughout Australia.

80. Are there any practical lessons to be learned from the 1918 pandemic?

Looking back at how U.S. cities coped during the pandemic, researchers have discovered that municipalities imposing the most stringent containment measures fared better than their counterparts whose plans were cobbled together far too late in the course of the infection's spread. Ordering citizens to wear masks, limiting public gatherings, and imposing fines on those who flouted the rules were just a few of the measures taken to contain the highly contagious flu.

St. Louis, for example, fared far better than did Philadelphia, which was so hard hit that flu victims' bodies began piling up because quarantine measures came too late. So many people were sickened or died, Philadelphia's public health infrastructure was strained. Analyzing the containment measures used during the pandemic offers many lessons for today's public health authorities. (See **Figure 7**).

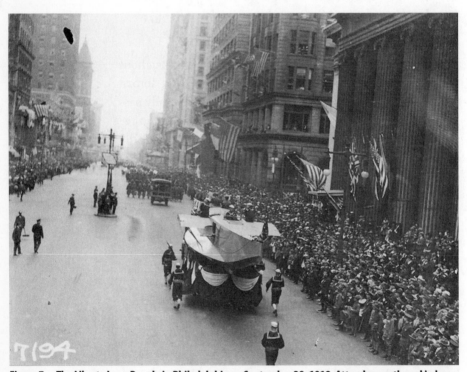

Figure 7 The Liberty Loan Parade in Philadelphia on September 28, 1918. Attendees gathered in huge numbers, and a few days later the city was stricken with one of the worst outbreaks in the country.
Courtesy of Naval Historical Center.

In two unusual studies published in 2007, 21st-century researchers have found that nonpharmaceutical efforts imposed during the deadly 1918 flu season probably spared thousands of lives. Indeed, quarantine measures and other steps taken to prevent infection in 1918 still have relevancy today and can be used in the event a sweeping flu pandemic should again occur. By looking back into America's public health past, investigators discovered that cities imposing strict quarantine rules immediately after the first local cases were reported reduced their death rates by up to half. It took nearly a century for these simple facts to come to light.

Across the United States, public health officials closed schools, theaters, churches, and dance halls—any place where large numbers of people were likely to congregate. St. Louis introduced several containment measures within 2 days of the first reported cases. But even though Philadelphia, Boston, and New Orleans imposed similar measures, they took much longer to implement them, and as a result, more people died.

Some cities, such as Kansas City, Missouri, went beyond common measures of quarantine and made it more difficult for people to gather. Public health authorities there took the additional step of banning weddings and funerals if more than 20 people were expected. Seattle's mayor ordered all citizens to wear gauze facemasks (see **Figure 8**); public health authorities in New York City and other large population centers nationwide issued similar orders. In New York City, which had one of the most authoritarian public health agencies in the world, yearlong jail terms were imposed on anyone caught coughing or sneezing in public. Days after the law took effect, courtrooms and jails began to fill with dozens of the guilty.

The New York City Department of Health held enormous sway over its citizens in the early 1900s and is perhaps best known for banning Mary Mallon, the notorious Typhoid Mary, to North Brother Island in 1915. North Brother is one

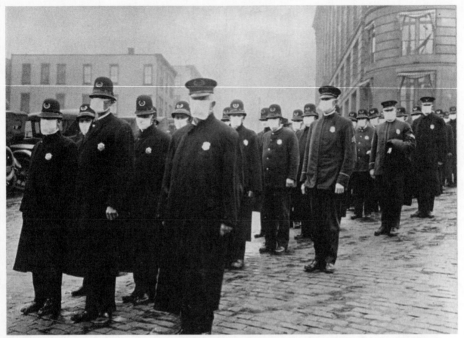

Figure 8   Policemen in Seattle wearing masks made by the Red Cross during the influenza epidemic, December 1918. Officials feared mass hysteria in major cities. Citizens were urged to stay indoors and avoid congested areas. Here, policemen patrol the streets to ensure public safety.
Courtesy of National Archives, photo no. 165-WW-269B-25.

of several quarantine islands off the city's coast. Mallon remained there until her death in 1938. Deemed a public health menace for infecting 47 people with typhoid during her years as a cook, city health authorities thought it best to minimize any threat by keeping Mary, quite literally, at bay.

Many flu sufferers and some people thought to have the flu (but perhaps who did not) were also banned to one or another of New York City's quarantine islands, a chain of tiny islets in the East River. (The islands are part of a dark New York past when quarantine was imposed because effective antimicrobials did not exist.) Yet New York was not alone in its aggressive stance against influenza. Chicago was also very strict, banning spitting and threatening to arrest anyone caught sneezing in public.

In 2007, a large collaborative team conducted one of two illuminating studies of the era. Investigators from the National Institute of Allergy and Infectious Diseases, the Department of Veterans Affairs, and Harvard University's School of Public Health examined how 17 U.S. cities fared in the fall of 1918. The researchers found a definite correlation between the number of interventions imposed and resulting death rate by the pandemic's end. The second study, which was conducted by British investigators at Imperial College London, examined the fate of 16 American cities and zeroed in on the start and stop dates of interventions imposed to curtail infections.

Timing when to impose and when to lift interventions was important in determining who lived or died in the pandemic. Cities that lifted their protective measures too soon saw a rise in the infection rate and a need to reimpose quarantines and other efforts. Using modern computer modeling, Dr. Neil Ferguson of the Imperial College found that San Francisco had the most effective protective measures of the 16 cities he and his colleagues studied. The team estimates the death rate there would have been 25% higher had public health officials not initiated interventions when they did. However, Ferguson's mathematical modeling also revealed that had San Francisco left containment measures in place from September 1918 through May 1919, deaths might have been reduced even more.

In a modern assault against a pandemic flu strain public health authorities would turn to vaccines and antiviral medications, two weapons that did not exist when the world fought a lethal form of influenza that killed millions of people.

Without such medical interventions, public health authorities in 1918 had to be more creative in their efforts to protect populations. Many turned to strategies that experts say would still be relevant in a 21st-century fight against pandemic flu. In a critique of the research, Dr. Anthony Fauci, director of the National Institute of Allergy and Infectious Diseases, says lessons from the two studies are important for pandemic planning today. Many of the strategies, such as limiting public gatherings, can help minimize infections in the event of another devastating flu outbreak.

81. Was the 1918 flu caused by a bird virus?

In 2005, scientists confirmed that a bird flu virus caused the 1918 influenza pandemic. The pathogen apparently jumped the species barrier directly from birds to humans—an extraordinarily unusual occurrence. Prior to the collaborative effort of many laboratories, which illuminated this fact, scientists had no idea why the 1918 strain was so incredibly lethal. Years of research went into studies that allowed medical investigators to draw the conclusion.

As part of the research, a team at the Armed Forces Institute of Pathology in Washington, D.C., identified viral molecules in the lung tissue of an Alaska Native woman who died of the flu in 1918. Her body had been preserved in the Alaskan permafrost. Additionally, the researchers studied fragments of the virus that had infected two U.S. Army soldiers who also died of influenza the same year. The soldiers' specimens had been preserved in the institute's vast repository of tissue samples. In each instance, investigators found infinitesimal pieces of the viral puzzle. Remains of the pathogen retrieved from the samples were not infectious. But the telltale fragments revealed enough molecular evidence that, ultimately, scientists at the Centers for Disease Control and Prevention were able to resurrect the deadly pathogen in a laboratory.

How scientists learned that a bird virus jumped the species barrier is a lesson in the remarkable nature of medical detective work. Researchers were able to determine from the genetics of the virus that it had crossed from birds to people in a single leap, and they were able to identify the specific genes in the virus that made it so exceptionally lethal. Neither the 1957

Asian flu nor the 1968 Hong Kong flu were nearly as deadly, and the latter two viruses didn't jump directly from birds.

Efforts at the pathology institute involving the pioneering work of Drs. Jeffrey Taubenberger and Ann Reid consumed nearly a decade. Later in the series of analyses, scientists at Mt. Sinai School of Medicine in New York City and the CDC joined the research.

Taubenberger and Reid were able to identify the genes of the 1918 influenza virus based on specimens from the three flu victims. Dr. Christopher Basler of Mt. Sinai studied the molecular blueprint of the virus, and using it like a recipe, began re-creating the basic molecular building blocks of the 1918 strain in the lab. "The main goals of the work were to understand why the 1918 flu was so deadly," Basler told the Long Island New York newspaper *Newsday*.

Working with Drs. Adolfo Garcia-Sastre and Peter Palese of Mount Sinai, Basler created plasmids, a tiny circular loop of genes. The scientists then shipped the plasmids to the CDC where they were insinuated into human lung cells. Within days they emerged as full-blown replicas of the 1918 virus. Dr. Terrence Tumpey led the final and most critical steps—reconstruction of the killer strain (see **Figure 9**). He underscored that the work was conducted in a BSL-3 high-containment laboratory where every precaution was taken to prevent viral escape.

The step-by-step procedures undertaken by scientists to identify and reconstruct a virus that murdered millions around the globe were reported in elaborate detail in two scientific papers published simultaneously in separate journals. And because they essentially provided a recipe for resurrecting one of the most pervasive killers of all time, leading public health officials released a statement underlining national and international security concerns. "Some [scientists] have understandably

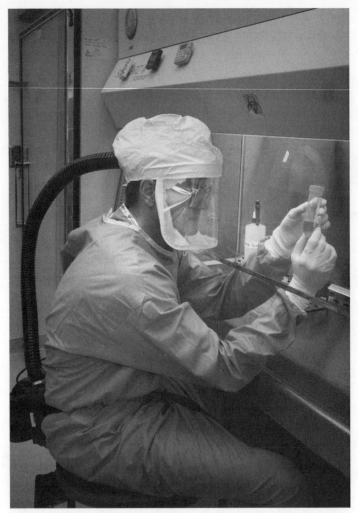

Figure 9   Dr. Terrence Tumpey working in a BSL-3 lab with a reconstructed version of the 1918 flu virus.
Courtesy of the Centers for Disease Control and Prevention.

questioned whether these research findings should be reported in scientific journals because of concern that this knowledge could be used by those with nefarious intent," wrote Drs. Julie Gerberding of the CDC and Anthony Fauci of the National Institute of Allergy and Infectious Diseases. "Prior to publication, these scientific papers were reviewed by the

National Science Advisory Board for Biosecurity (NSABB), an advisory committee to the U.S. Secretary of Health and Human Services and to the heads of all federal departments and agencies that conduct or support life science research."

The NSABB unanimously decided the reports were critically important to the scientific community and laid the ground-work for a fuller understanding of flu viruses that jump the species barrier. Such knowledge, according to the NSABB, also can aid the scientific and medical communities in the development of diagnostic tests, antiviral medications, and vaccines.

82. How was the 1918 flu virus retrieved from an Alaska Native woman?

To Dr. Johan Hultin, a retired San Francisco pathologist, the cause of the 1918 flu was the ultimate medical mystery. Even after scientists learned in the 1930s that a virus caused the pandemic, there were still countless questions that persisted for many decades. Hultin first trekked to the Arctic Circle in the early 1950s, searching for answers that he believed were buried—and preserved—in the graves of Alaska Natives who died in the pandemic. Theory held that traces of the viral killer probably remained in suspended animation deep in the lungs of victims buried below layers of ice.

In 1997, when Hultin learned of a project under way at the Armed Forces Institute of Pathology, where scientists were trying to discover why so many people died at the close of World War I, he volunteered again to go to Alaska, offering to pay for his trip and supplies. Having familiarized himself with the people and the terrain nearly a half century earlier, Hultin was eager to go. Indeed, the intrepid Californian traveled solo to the Alaskan tundra in 1997, assuring the team of medical investigators at the pathology institute in Washington, D.C., that he knew of a mass grave that contained the bodies of 72 flu victims.

Hultin had embarked on his first expedition in 1951 while still a medical student at the University of Iowa. He went to Brevig Mission on Alaska's Seward Peninsula, hoping to obtain lung tissue from people buried in the permafrost. Hultin was inspired to embark on a virus hunt after a virologist who was visiting the University of Iowa mentioned that evidence of the killer strain was probably preserved in the frozen bodies of Alaska Natives. Medical historians say the small village of Brevig was devastated by the flu, which spared few of the villagers who lived there. The infection was passed person to person at warp speed in November 1918, nearly wiping out all of Brevig's residents.

In 1951, villagers gave Hultin permission to open a mass grave where he found intact bodies and was able to retrieve tissue samples, which he took back to his Iowa lab. Using techniques current during the early 1950s, he couldn't find a trace of the 1918 flu virus. Forty-six years later, however, there was a dramatic turning point. Again, he obtained permission to open the mass grave. Although he found only one intact body, that of a woman, he managed to obtain a sufficient lung tissue sample, which he sent to the Armed Forces Institute of Pathology. There, Drs. Jeffrey Taubenberger and Ann Reid were piecing together molecular evidence in an effort to unmask the 1918 killer. Hultin's contribution helped Taubenberger and Reid identify the pathogen's genes.

83. What are some of the theories about the origin of the great pandemic?

Some contemporary theorists suggest the most fully described "start" of the 1918 flu are the Fort Riley military cases, which flared in the spring of 1918. Fort Riley at the time was a vast Army base in the heart of Kansas. It was a major training site as U.S. military recruits were readied for war. Yet other theories point to the flu's start years before 1918 and thousands of miles away from Kansas. One prominent theory posits that the flu's epicenter was indeed at a military encampment, but a British one located in France where military doctors at the time kept fastidious records on a mysterious outbreak.

You may ask why some theorists believe the flu began in Kansas. The medical literature reveals that dozens upon dozens of young recruits who were being trained for the war effort were assigned to Fort Riley, and it wasn't long after their arrival at the sprawling base that many would contract a respiratory illness. Soldiers were crowded in barracks, which made transmission of a virus not just possible but very likely. The soldiers then carried the infection with them, wherever they were sent. From Fort Riley, the flu is believed to have fanned out to other parts of the United States before making its way around the globe.

What may seem to be a likely starting point of the infection actually may be the most accurate description of the pandemic's first wave, the one in the spring of 1918. Yes, the outbreak at Fort Riley was serious—and pervasive—but the death toll was nowhere near the more highly virulent second and third waves that began months later. Could the flu have been brought into Fort Riley from elsewhere? Twenty-first-century theories suggest, yes, that is not only possible but quite likely.

Fort Riley military doctors documented respiratory illnesses sweeping through the massive compound beginning in March 1918. Shortly afterward, the same sickness was being documented elsewhere in the United States, especially in New York, Philadelphia, and Boston. In retrospect, some scientists now believe the illnesses in the spring were clearly a harbinger of what was to come in the fall.

But just as some theorists accept the idea that the pandemic got its start in Kansas in 1918, others have followed differing lines of evidence. Researchers who've dug deeper and looked harder for the elusive origins of the 1918 flu say the medical literature contains strong hints of an even earlier start. Sporadic outbreaks of respiratory illnesses were reported as early as 1915 in the United States, suggestive of a virus that had not yet fully become a pandemic strain. And as intriguing as that notion may seem, still other theorists suggest the origins of the deadly pandemic may not have been in the United States at all.

Influential British virologist Dr. John Oxford agrees that the flu didn't emerge suddenly in 1918. He uncovered evidence implicating an earlier date: 1916—in France. Oxford's theory comes as a result of studying medical data appearing in the venerable British medical journal *The Lancet*. Thumbing through a 1916 edition, he believes he stumbled upon the first documented evidence of the respiratory illness that would become known as the deadly influenza.

In *The Lancet*, British military doctors wrote about a highly contagious respiratory illness in 1916, which they called infectious purulent bronchitis that affected troops stationed in Etaples, France. They found that 50% of the soldiers who contracted infectious purulent bronchitis died of the infection. Up to 40,000 British soldiers were processed through the French base, according to Oxford, prior to being deployed to the trenches where Great Britain fought Germany.

Military physicians writing at the time in *The Lancet* described a condition that was far deadlier than the Germans' bullets because of the toll the illness took on otherwise healthy troops.

The infection spread quickly and easily throughout the Etaples encampment. Infectious purulent bronchitis caused soldiers' skin to darken, which contemporary experts say is a direct result of oxygen deprivation. Soldiers' lungs were so ravaged by what medical investigators now believe was a cytokine storm—the highly charged immune system attack—that doctors who conducted the autopsies nearly a century ago were shocked by what they saw. Experts now believe the flu played a role in ending World War I because an increasing number of soldiers were too sick to fight.

Oxford is convinced that *The Lancet* report is the most descriptive explanation of the beginnings of an infection that became known interchangeably as the Spanish flu and the killer grippe. All told, the 1916 study contained a 145-case sampling. Perhaps the most eye-opening revelation in the report is the persistence of a smoldering illness that never left the base. It continued to affect new groups of fresh recruits no matter how well the barracks were scrubbed.

In an interview with the newspaper *Newsday*, Oxford said mortality statistics from the 1916 medical report are strikingly similar to figures today involving human cases of bird flu. The fatality rate for humans who contract bird flu, usually as a direct result of contact with bird droppings or through handling sick fowl, is about 50%. And so it was among British soldiers in 1916.

Regardless of which retelling you accept—whether the 1918 flu began in Kansas or at a British Army base in France— there is no denying that the 1918 flu continues to be of academic and scientific importance today. Experts say the pandemic offers numerous lessons about what it is like when every human life on the planet is under threat from a single virus.

Oxford sees parallels between contemporary bird flu and what appeared to be the beginnings of an influenza outbreak that exploded in 1918. The world "is long overdue for a virus like H5N1 to take off," he told the newspaper. "Certainly another pandemic can occur." "The World Health Organization and the United Nations are both in agreement with that."

84. How did people respond to quarantine measures?

Most people throughout the United States and elsewhere followed the rapidly developed plans announced by public health officials. In some instances, the sick and all their household members were not to leave their homes. In most instances, though, quarantine simply meant restricting the movement of people to prevent as many as possible from coming in contact with someone who might be infected.

There was, however, a key problem with instituting quarantine measures, a fact many municipalities quickly discovered in 1918: Officials often called for quarantines only after an outbreak was under way. Still, quarantine was, and still is, a highly effective method of preventing the spread of a contagious disease. When infected people are isolated from those who are healthy, and when public health authorities restrict the movement and gatherings of individuals, then disease transmission patterns can be broken.

Quarantine measures were not a highly unusual intrusion into the lives of Americans in 1918. Restrictive measures were already very familiar to people who had experienced quarantines instituted during outbreaks of measles, typhoid, smallpox, and other highly contagious infections. Moreover, in an era that lacked the sophisticated pharmaceuticals in existence today, public health officials had few other options to limit the flu's spread. Quarantine measures involved not only closing theaters, libraries, and other public places, but also meant setting curfews that kept people off city streets.

Public health officials learned an extraordinary lesson as a result of the pandemic: When a highly virulent and easily transmissible infection is spreading, quarantine measures have to be far more expansive—and restrictive. In 1918, public health authorities quickly ordered additional measures of containment in some areas, calling for thousands of gauze masks. Volunteers, including those working through local Red Cross affiliates, began sewing facial protectors around the clock. Despite the urgency, some people balked at having to cover their noses and mouths with the masks. In cities such as Seattle, passengers were ordered off trolleys or were refused to board unless they were wearing one.

PART EIGHT

21st-Century Pandemic Planning

Is there a nationwide pandemic flu plan in
the United States?

Does the U.S. government have "quarantine powers"
even when there isn't a pandemic?

Should families and individuals develop
their own pandemic flu plans?

More . . .

85. Is there a nationwide pandemic flu plan in the United States?

The U.S. government announced its pandemic flu preparedness plan in November 2005. Anyone can read the plan, which is accessible online at www.hhs.gov/pandemicflu/plan. According to the document's wording, the plan is based on a simple premise: "Once a pandemic is triggered by the emergence of a novel influenza A subtype, it is a global event and all countries are at risk."

The lengthy and highly detailed plan leaves no stone unturned. It calls for immediately ramping up surveillance to track viral spread and calls for collaborative containment measures with states and other countries. Additionally, the document calls for stockpiling antiviral medications and vaccines, and working with the pharmaceutical industry to expand the production of both. A final major component involves putting into effect a major communications effort that will keep the public informed.

86. Do individual states also have pandemic flu plans?

All U.S. states have individual pandemic flu preparedness plans, which take into account a wide variety of factors to protect their populations. Each state's lead health agency has posted its pandemic flu preparedness plan online, and it is probably a good idea for residents in each state to familiarize themselves with the major bullet points of the plans. The plans are essentially blueprints for action and can double as strategies for other major medical emergencies.

State health departments list a range of concerns that might arise in the event of pandemic influenza and outline how those issues would be addressed. They also caution that it may be difficult to receive medical care and that services and supplies may be limited. For example, as part of their preplanning, states have already determined how many mechanical ventilators are available in each county or region. The equipment is vital in the event of severe influenza because mechanical ventilators aid patients in respiratory distress. A federal ventilator stockpile exists. However, in a flu disaster on the scale of the 1918 pandemic, many states probably would not have enough of the devices to meet demand. Some state pandemic planners say that rationing ventilators could become reality should a severe flu pandemic occur. Healthcare professionals would have to decide which of their ailing patients would receive the aid of the device.

Surveillance is another major focus of state pandemic plans, and all underscore (as a top priority) the need to quickly identify areas of concentrated flu activity—hot zones—and control further spread. Essential to an effective public health response is a sufficient number of medical personnel to meet as much of the demand for care as possible. Bear in mind that during a major emergency, you can't expect hospitals and other medical facilities to function as usual. The state of Maine's Center for Disease Control and Prevention points out in the introduction to its plan that "a number of healthcare workers and first responders available to work will be reduced because of illness or needing to care for family members; and basic resources could be limited." To help alleviate problems associated with staffing, some states, such as New York, suggest calling retired doctors and nurses into duty.

As with all states, the California preparedness plan emphasizes that control and containment of influenza will involve medical and nonmedical strategies, including "isolation, quarantine, infection control, antiviral treatment and prophylaxis, and if available, vaccination." The plan also calls for tracking and responding to secondary influenza waves.

87. If vaccination is the leading method of flu prevention, why isn't it the only strategy needed in a pandemic?

Given current manufacturing methods it might take months to produce a sufficient supply of flu vaccines to meet the needs of millions of people. That is why additional methods of prevention may be necessary. Vaccine production is tedious. Apart from time-consuming manufacturing techniques that involve chicken eggs, production would be labored by the sheer number of doses required to address the needs of millions of people. Vaccine manufacturers would be more than doubling their current output for seasonal vaccines. Even though advanced production techniques that do not rely on eggs could shave some time off production, there probably would be a perception of laboriousness in an atmosphere that certainly would be ruled by panic and fear.

88. Why would quarantine measures be part of 21st-century pandemic flu preparedness plans?

Quarantine is only one measure among many that would be employed in the event of a major flu disaster. Quarantine has more than one definition. In one sense, it could mean isolating people who are infected with a deadly flu strain to prevent further spread of the flu. It also means that in the midst of an outbreak, healthy individuals' freedom of movement is restrained to prevent contact with, and spread of, the flu virus.

89. Does the U.S. government have "quarantine powers" even when there isn't a pandemic?

The Centers for Disease Control and Prevention, a U.S. federal health agency, has in recent years increased the number of its U.S. Quarantine Stations, which are located in airports and along land-border crossings nationwide. The 20 stations are integral to the nation's pandemic disease defense, protecting U.S. citizens from infectious conditions that might otherwise be carried into the country. For example, when an international flight lands with a sick passenger onboard, health officers from a U.S. Quarantine Station have legal authority to evaluate the individual.

Officers are trained in the diagnosis of exotic infections and also possess legal authority to detain a passenger with unusual symptoms. An ailing passenger would be kept in the station only long enough for a thorough medical evaluation before being released or sent to an isolation unit at a hospital. The CDC has increased the number of health officers as a way of bolstering the defense against imported infections. According to the agency, there is a hit list of infections that it actively works to keep at bay. These infectious disorders include cholera, diphtheria, infectious tuberculosis, plague, smallpox, yellow fever, and viral hemorrhagic fevers. SARS was added in April 2003 and new types of flu that can trigger a pandemic were added in 2005.

In the event of a pandemic, the network of quarantine stations is expected to play a key role, acting as a firewall to keep the infection out of the United States, and when necessary, coordinating wide-ranging plans that, again, can include evaluation and detention. The stations are not equipped, however, to isolate entire planeloads of passengers.

90. Is port-of-entry quarantine a relatively new idea?

The first quarantine station and hospital in the United States were built in Philadelphia in 1799 following a sweeping yellow fever epidemic 6 years earlier. Yellow fever is a viral illness carried by mosquitoes, and the deadly epidemic claimed the lives of about 4,000 people in what was then the largest city in the United States. In the late 18th century, Philadelphia was the seat of the federal government, and the outbreak was so horrific that George Washington was among those forced to flee until the illnesses subsided. The outbreak awakened a young nation to a need for quarantine as a way to protect itself from infectious diseases. In 1878, the National Quarantine Act was approved, which transferred quarantine powers from states to the federal government.

91. Should families and individuals develop their own pandemic flu plans?

Pandemic flu planners strongly urge families to develop their own plan for a major medical emergency, such as global influenza. As part of its extensive pandemic flu plan, the state of Washington has published a brochure that focuses on what individuals can do to prepare for a flu pandemic. The brochure is published in English, Spanish, Chinese, Russian, and Vietnamese and can be downloaded from the Internet by logging on to the following address: *www.doh.wa.gov/panflu/ pdf/PanfluPocket.pdf.*

Here are a few tips from the brochure: Individuals developing a household pandemic plan should maintain at least a week's worth of food and water for each family member. For anyone who takes medication for a chronic disorder, the brochure recommends having a week's supply on hand as part of effective pandemic planning. Families also should maintain items to relieve flu symptoms, such as ibuprofen and acetaminophen for fever, cold packs, blankets, extra water, and fruit juice. Keeping a cell phone handy is considered a plus.

PART NINE

Guarding Your Health

Seasonal flu arrives every year and someone in my office always gets sick. What is the best way to protect myself?

Are there additional steps that I can take to prevent catching the flu?

Is stockpiling your own antiviral medications a good idea?

More . . .

92. *Seasonal flu arrives every year and someone in my office always gets sick. What is the best way to protect myself?*

Vaccination is your best defense against seasonal flu and many companies offer annual flu vaccinations for employees at little or no cost. If your workplace does not provide the service, you might want to jot down your thoughts and drop the idea in the company suggestion box. Company-sponsored flu vaccinations are a surefire way to reduce wintertime absenteeism when everyone participates. If your company does not have an onsite nurse who is licensed to administer flu vaccines, there are companies that provide annual flu vaccinations for companies of all sizes. Costs for administering vaccinations are offset by continued productivity during a time of year when many people might be absent as a result of the flu. Moreover, when vaccinations are made available, companies can benefit from the old cliché: An ounce of prevention is worth a pound of cure.

93. *Are there additional steps that I can take to prevent catching the flu?*

Along with taking advantage of flu vaccination, you can take several simple steps to reduce your chances of infection. Earlier we mentioned the importance of **hand hygiene**. This refers to washing your hands during the course of your day, or at least keeping a dispenser of an alcohol-based hand sanitizer available. Healthcare providers suggest washing (in warm water with soap) for at least 15 seconds. Hand washing is important because many people unwittingly touch their faces unaware that pathogens can be introduced through their mouths, noses, or even by rubbing their eyes.

hand hygiene
Frequent hand washing, or at the very least, frequent use of a hand sanitizer to prevent self-infection or passing infections along to others.

Even though hand washing is a seemingly low-tech method of protection, it is one of the most overlooked. The Centers for Disease Control and Prevention notes that apart from being vaccinated, the simple act of hand washing is the single most important method of preventing the spread of viral and bacterial infections.

94. Okay, the term hand hygiene makes perfect sense. But what does cough hygiene mean?

Again, this is something your parents probably cautioned you about many times as a child, but of course, they probably didn't use the fancy **cough hygiene** terminology, or its equally arcane cousin—cough etiquette. These terms simply mean cover your mouth when you cough. This is important advice wherever you are—at home, school, at the mall, or in the workplace because inattention to *how* you cough could result in many people around you getting sick if you have the flu.

If you're curious about the basics of "Cough Etiquette 101." here are few simple tips:

1. Cover your nose and mouth with a tissue every time you cough and appropriately dispose the tissue. Do not leave it lying around.
2. If you do not have a tissue, cough into your sleeve.
3. Always wash your hands after coughing.
4. Stay home when you are sick.

Just as these simple guidelines should be followed for seasonal flu, many states have included similar information on the importance of cough hygiene (or etiquette) in their pandemic flu preparedness plan. They believe that in the event of an influenza disaster, individuals who pay attention to how they cough are less likely to spread the infection.

95. Is stockpiling my own antiviral medications a good idea?

Physicians and public health agencies emphasize that stock-piling medications such as oseltamivir and zanamivir is not

cough hygiene
Taking precaution when ill with a respiratory condition to cover a cough with a tissue and to properly dispose of it after use.

only a bad idea, it is brazenly irresponsible behavior. Of course, health agencies stockpile antiviral medications in the event of a large-scale epidemic or pandemic. But these entities also employ professionals who are mindful of rotating medications into and out of their drug caches because they are keenly aware of expiration dates and issues of drug potency.

With the sale of prescription drugs over the Internet, it is becoming increasingly simpler for individuals to consider developing their own medication stockpiles. It happened in New York City in 2001 involving the antibiotic ciprofloxa-cin—Cipro—in the wake of the anthrax scare. Many people nudged physicians to write prescriptions. But drug hoarders are often unaware of many underlying issues involving antivi-ral medications. Who knows whether you will ever develop a condition that can be treated with the drug you've stockpiled? What about the expiration date, or allergies to the drug? What about potential side effects or overdoses? There are too many unknowns and too many opportunities for something to go wrong. Do not start your own antiviral stockpile.

96. I've heard that getting enough sleep helps prevent the flu. Is that true?

Getting enough sleep is part of several simple measures you can take to remain healthy. The others include eating healthy foods, getting plenty of exercise, and reducing levels of stress. Each of these steps plays an integral role in healthy living and helps boost your immunity. Certainly, you would not rely on them alone as your defense against influenza. But when these measures are pursued along with several others (outlined in Questions 92 and 93 in greater detail) you can help minimize your odds of catching the flu while maximizing your overall state of health.

97. Should pregnant women get a flu shot? What about nursing mothers?

The flu shot is recommended for pregnant women, but the nasal spray vaccine is not advised because it is what is known as a live-attenuated influenza vaccine, or LAIV. Such vaccines are made up of weakened influenza viruses, the same three strains that are in flu shots. It is important that pregnant women consider a flu shot because observational studies suggest the illness is more severe in pregnant women, as are most viral illnesses. Whereas the flu may last a few days in a young, healthy woman who is not pregnant, the infection may last much longer in someone who is expecting. There is also an increased risk of pneumonia. Some doctors attribute the lengthier course of illness in pregnant women to their somewhat less robust immune system. If you are pregnant, you can ask for a thimerosal-free flu shot, especially if you are concerned about preservative use in vaccines. Vaccination does not pose a risk to pregnancy.

The Centers for Disease Control and Prevention notes that flu vaccination poses no known risks to breastfeeding mothers or their infants. There is a caveat for women who are allergic to eggs and who previously never had flu shots. Because eggs are involved in the production of vaccine doses, the potential for an allergic reaction exists. You should discuss flu vaccination with your physician, who needs to be aware of your medical history, before the injection is administered. Also, there are no contraindications against being immunized with the inhaled vaccine—the nasal spray—sold as FluMist if you are breastfeeding.

98. When you catch the flu why is it important to remain hydrated?

Fever is one of the characteristics of influenza and as a result can lead to dehydration. You don't need to purchase fancy hydration drinks (some of which are marketed specifically for the flu) because water often suffices. Some doctors suggest ice chips, juice, or soft fruits (such as melon slices) to maintain hydration.

99. How can I protect myself from bird flu?

Avian influenza—bird flu—is primarily a threat to birds and the chances of people coming in contact with the pathogen in Western countries are quite low, if not zero. Remember, avian flu is just that, a plague among birds. Most human infections have occurred in those parts of Asia, particularly Southeast Asia, where the population lives in close proximity with domestic fowl. Farmers in these countries have a greater chance of coming in contact with sick birds and/or their feces. Infections documented outside of Asia (Turkey is an example) also involved people who have had direct contact with sick birds. The avian outbreak has caused severe economic hardships in underdeveloped countries. Some families' entire flock is ordered destroyed after government inspectors find evidence of the infection in only one or two birds.

100. Should I stop eating chicken to avoid bird flu?

Your chances of coming in contact with the bird flu virus through the U.S. food supply are virtually nil. In the United States, the U.S. Department of Agriculture (USDA) is in charge of inspecting chickens at slaughterhouses and has strict guidelines about keeping sick birds with any kind of illness out of the food supply.

Granted, common bacteria, such as *Salmonella* and *Campylobacter*, are often found in raw poultry sold in supermarkets. You can protect yourself from these pathogens by properly handling raw poultry and making certain you cook the meat thoroughly. Cooking poultry at a temperature of 165° Fahrenheit ensures that microbes are destroyed. Consumer experts strongly encourage the use of a thermometer to determine when the meat reaches the optimum temperature while cooking.

If for some unforeseen reason the virtually impossible occurs and bird flu happens to have infected poultry that you've purchased, following the steps outlined for killing the two previously mentioned bacteria will also destroy the flu pathogen.

The USDA has developed consumer literature outlining the multiple barriers that have been put in place to ensure that the U.S. poultry industry and the public are protected from avian influenza. The USDA emphasizes that the "common sense steps of food safety self-defense" provide consumers with protection against any range of pathogens that can affect chickens and other fowl.

Appendix

Affiliated Physicians

Provides flu shots for businesses during flu season. Affiliated Physicians estimates that American businesses experience productivity losses during flu season as a result of sick workers. The company also carries a wealth of information on its website about avian influenza and how corporations can brace for it.

Company's literature states: "Beyond the human toll, influenza also results in a huge indirect economic loss for society, estimated to be as much as $20 billion annually. A CDC study shows that sick days and lost productivity can be decreased by 32 to 45 percent with flu vaccination of healthy working adults, thereby reducing the estimated $7 billion cost to American businesses alone."

18 East 48th Street
(at Madison Avenue)
2nd Floor
New York, NY 10017
212-935-8725
Toll Free: 877-292-5546
Fax: 212-935-2873
www.affiliatedphysicians.net

American Lung Association

Offers a wide range of information about the flu, including where to find clinics in your area providing flu shots. Sponsors *Faces of Influenza,* an educational website.

The purpose of the site is to "put a face on influenza in the United States and show firsthand the seriousness of this potentially deadly infectious disease."

61 Broadway, 6th Floor
NY, NY 10006 (Nat'l headquarters)
For Influenza Prevention Programs
Contact Your Local ALA Chapter
1-800-LUNG-USA
www.facesofinfluenza.org

Centers for Disease Control and Prevention

One of the world's elite centers for the study of viral pathogens and global surveillance for seasonal and exotic influenza strains. The CDC also carries a wealth of consumer-oriented information about influenza, which includes proven methods of preventing the spread of the infection. Many of the most important studies conducted on seasonal and pandemic flu strains have occurred at the CDC.

The agency was established in the late 1940s as a division of the U.S. Public Health Service and is based in Atlanta, Georgia. On a website devoted entirely to seasonal influenza, the agency carries information about flu vaccination, symptoms, antiviral medications, people at risk for complications, and how to care for yourself when you are ill with the flu.

The CDC has separate sites for avian, swine and pandemic influenza. CDC health officials emphasize on the site that between 5 and 20 percent of the U.S. population is sickened annually with the flu, more than 200,000 people are hospitalized and about 36,000 die of the condition.

1600 Clifton Road
Atlanta, GA 30333
1-800-CDC-INFO (800-232-4636)
1-888-232-6348 TTY
www.cdc.gov/flu

Families Fighting Flu

Organization developed by families whose children died or were severely sickened by the flu.

According to the organization's literature, it is a non-profit made up of families and pediatricians who have experienced first-hand what it is like to lose a child to the flu or to have a child experience severe medical complications from the flu. The organization was incorporated in 2005 with the mission of reducing pediatric deaths due to the flu by raising awareness about the importance of getting all children vaccinated against the flu. Members of the organization have regularly addressed the CDC's advisory committee on immunization practices, urging panelists to adopt comprehensive vaccination policies.

4201 Wilson Blvd.
Arlington, Va 22203
1-888-2ENDFLU
www.familiesfightingflu.org

FluWatch

Sponsored by Canada's national flu surveillance system and coordinated through the Centre for Infectious Disease Prevention and Control at the Public Health Agency of Canada. According to information provided by FluWatch, the program began in 1996 to provide "a national picture of influenza activity." The program has several goals:

1) Early detection of influenza activity in Canada.
2) Provision of timely and up-to-date information on flu activity in Canada and abroad to health professionals as well as the public.
3) Monitoring of circulating strains of influenza, including new sub-types and anti-viral resistance.
4) Contributing viral surveillance information to the World Health Organization.

The site carries a wealth of information about vaccination, travel, emergency preparedness and health promotion. The health agency itself has numerous regional offices throughout the country. Main branches are in Ontario and Manitoba.

Public Health Agency of Canada
130 Colonnade Road
A.L. 6501H
Ottawa, Ontario   K1A 0K9
and
1015 Arlington Street
Winnipeg, Manitoba   R3E 3R2
www.phac-aspc.gc.ca/fluwatch

FluWiki

Provides information on its website about avian influenza and the number of people affected by it. Statistics are based on figures compiled by the World Health Organization. Has a link to a comic book produced by King County health officials in the Seattle area, tilted "No Ordinary Flu." The illustrated book, which can be downloaded, is about the 1918 flu. The FluWiki site also carries information about pandemic preparedness and addresses national and international surveillance of suspect flu strains.
www.fluwikie.com

Immunization Action Coalition

Carries a wealth of information on its website about the flu under the title: Vaccine Information for the Public and Health Professionals.

The Immunization Action Coalition, a non-profit organization, works to increase immunization rates and prevent infectious disease.

1573 Selby Avenue
Suite. 234
St. Paul, MN 55104
651-647-9009
Fax: 651-647-9131
www.vaccineinformation.org/flu

Infectious Diseases Society of America

The organization is made up of physicians, scientists and public health officials who specialize in infectious diseases. Influenza is a major focus of the society, highlighted by its Pandemic and Seasonal Principles for U.S. Action. In terms of seasonal flu the society suggests that annual flu vaccination be made a requirement for all healthcare workers. Those who decline should do so in writing, stating religious, philosophical or medical reasons. A key tenet is using lessons learned to combat seasonal flu to prepare for the emergence of a pandemic strain. The principles also call for a pandemic influenza vaccine master program and an improvement in influenza diagnostic tools.

1300 Wilson Blvd
Suite 300
Arlington, VA 22209
Phone: 703-299-0200
Fax: 703-299-0204
www.idsociety.org

National Foundation for Infectious Diseases

Sponsors the Childhood Influenza Immunization Coalition, a group of 25 of the leading public health, medical, patient and parent groups in the United States. The foundation carries a large compendium of information on its website about the flu, vaccination, immunizing healthcare workers against the flu, general information about influenza for consumers and a variety of fact sheets about flu virus infection.

4733 Bethesda Avenue
Suite 750
Bethesda, MD 20814
Phone: 301-656-0003
Fax: 301-907-0878
www.nfid.org

National Institute for Allergy and Infectious Diseases

The institute is one of the 19 institutes of the National Institutes of Health (NIH). The NIH is an agency of the U.S. Department of Health and Human Services. The National Institute of Allergy and Infectious Diseases funded the Influenza Genome Sequencing Project to advance scientific knowledge of the flu and further the understanding of how flu viruses emerge, spread and cause epidemics. The institute's website devoted to influenza is one of the most comprehensive, covering subjects that range from flu transmission, symptoms and prevention to in-depth explanations of how flu viruses mutate and up-to-date reports on pandemic flu research.

ite also carries information about the 1918 flu pandemic and updates on the Centers of Excellence for Influenza Research and Surveillance. The centers allow the National Institute for Allergy and Infectious Diseases to expand nationally and internationally its surveillance of flu viruses in animals and support several priorities regarding the evolution and spread of influenza viruses. The institute's influenza site also carries a wealth of consumer-oriented information.

6610 Rockledge Drive, MSC 6612
Bethesda, MD 20892-6612
Toll-Free: 866-284-4107
Local: 301-496-5717
TDD: 800-877-8339 (for hearing impaired)
Fax: 301-402-3573
www.niaid.nih.gov/topics/flu

PandemicFlu.gov

Bills itself as the "one-stop access" for information about pandemic influenza. The site carries updated information about avian flu as well as the U.S. Pandemic Influenza Preparedness Plan. Individual state pandemic flu strategies can be accessed through the site. The latest information on vaccine research, the use of masks and antiviral medications also can be found on the site.

Photos, statistics and information about the 1918 pandemic have been compiled to acquaint visitors to the website with the largest and most lethal infectious disease outbreak in history. PandemicFlu. gov is sponsored by the U.S. Department of Health and Human Services.

www.pandemicflu.gov

United Nations
Among the leading agencies worldwide keeping track of bird flu outbreaks and the implications for human health (See World Health Organization). The U.N. regularly holds news conferences to keep the public abreast of outbreaks of avian influenza in birds and what those outbreaks mean for people nearby and elsewhere in the world. The U.N. maintains a website titled **Avian Influenza and the Pandemic Threat**. The information is available in multiple languages, including Arabic, Russian, Chinese, French and Spanish, to name a few.

www.un-influenza.org

U.S. Food and Drug Administration
The FDA plays a major role nationally and internationally in the determination of strains to be included in each year's seasonal flu vaccine. But the agency role goes much farther. The FDA not only is the agency that approved the drugs used to combat the flu, it also is the agency that monitors its effects and calls for action – if needed – when antivirals trigger untoward effects. The FDA's influenza websites on influenza are among the most comprehensive in the world. The agency makes note each year when the vaccine for the upcoming flu season is approved; it reports inspections of vaccine manufacturers' facilities; warns the public about fraudulent flu-fighting products, and provides information for health care providers on the annual flu-vaccine supply.

In addition, the FDA has consumer-oriented information about flu symptoms, treatment, vaccination and the use of antiviral medications. Its Flu Fact Sheet capsulizes many common questions consumers have about the flu:

1) How does one catch the flu?
2) Who is most at risk?
3) What are the signs of the flu?
4) How well does the flu shot work?

5) Are there drugs to treat it?

6) What should I do if I get the flu?

Every year experts from the FDA, World Health Organization, CDC and other health agencies around the world study virus samples collected globally in an effort to identify strains that may cause the most illness in the upcoming season.

5600 Fishers Lane

Rockville, MD 20857-0001

1-888-463-6332

www.fda.gov/oc/opacom/hottopics/flu.html

World Health Organization (WHO)

A major global health agency that plays a leading role in the identification of seasonal flu strains and maintains surveillance of avian strains circulating worldwide. WHO is a specialized agency of the United Nations, and its main role is to combat diseases, especially infectious ones that can crop up anywhere in the world.

The agency has been in the vanguard of those tracking the advancement of avian influenza around the world and taking note of human cases of the infection. It maintains a timeline on its website of all major events involving H5N1, the bird flu strain under surveillance as it spreads through flocks of birds worldwide. The timeline also makes note of human cases and fatalities.

WHO also sponsors FluNet, a web page that is the cornerstone of the agency's global flu program, providing consumer-friendly information about influenza. WHO's web-based information is available in multiple languages.

Avenue Appia 20

1211 Geneva 27

Switzerland

1+ 41-22-791-2111

Fax: 1-41-22-791-3111

Telex: 415 416

Telegraph: UNISANTE GENEVA

www.who.int

Glossary

A

A influenza: *(See Type A, B, C influenza)*

Acute respiratory distress syndrome (ARDS): Sometimes simply referred to as respiratory distress syndrome. The National Heart, Lung, and Blood Institute notes that ARDS can occur as a result of infections, injuries, or other conditions that cause the lung's capillaries to leak more fluid than normal into the alveoli, the air sacs of the lungs. This prevents the lungs from filling with air and moving enough oxygen into the bloodstream.

Adamantanes: A class of antiviral medications capable of relieving flu symptoms. The two drugs in this class are amantadine (Symmetrel) and rimantadine (Flumadine). These drugs are effective only against Type A strains of influenza. Widespread resistance to this class of drugs in some parts of the world forced U.S. health officials to issue an embargo against their use until evidence surfaced that resistance was no longer a problem.

Adenovirus: A family of about 40 DNA viruses known to cause human infections, including the common cold.

Amantadine: A prescription medication licensed by drug regulators worldwide to relieve symptoms of influenza. Amantadine is an antiviral drug. Surprisingly, the medication also relieves the rigidity of Parkinson's disease.

Antibody: A Y-shaped protein that is made by the body's immune system in response to invasive foreign substances such as bacteria, viruses, protozoa, fungi, toxins, and even transplanted organs. Antibodies bind to specific molecules (antigens) on the surfaces of invasive bacteria, viruses, fungi, etc., to neutralize them.

Antigen: Any foreign substance that, when introduced into the body, stimulates an immune response, causing the body to release antibodies.

Antigenic drift: Continuous genetic-driven change that causes slight alterations on the surface of flu viruses at the site where antibodies bind. These changes allow flu viruses to outfox the body's immune system, necessitating the need for annual flu vaccinations. Antigenic drift occurs in both Type A and B influenza viruses. Antigenic drift facilitates the survival of flu viruses and their annual spread throughout populations.

Antigenic shift: A sudden, dramatic genetic change in a dominant circulating Type A influenza virus. The change results in surface antigens that have never before challenged the human immune system. The virus is produced through a recombination of genes. For example, when a particularly lethal strain that infects only animals jumps directly to a human, the result can be a pandemic strain that is easily transmitted person-to-person. Antigenic shifts occurred before each of the three pandemics that killed millions of people in the 20th century.

Attenuated vaccine: A vaccine made up of bacteria or viruses of the infection that is to be prevented through vaccination. An attenuated vaccine is one in which the microbe has been made less virulent through exposure to heat, chemicals or other processes.

Avian influenza: (*See bird flu*)

B

B influenza: (*See Type A, B, C influenza*)

Bacteria: A vast group of microscopic organisms ubiquitous throughout the world, many of which live on and within humans. The word is plural for bacterium. Bacteria multiply through fission or by forming spores. Bacteria and viruses are completely unrelated. Bacteria can be cultured in cell-free media in the laboratory, but viruses always require a host. People who are hospitalized for the flu often have secondary bacterial infections. Secondary bacterial infections are a leading cause of pneumonia in people severely sickened by the flu.

Bird flu: Influenza in wild aquatic birds. Type A influenza viruses are endemic to wild birds and thrive in their intestines. The viruses cause no disease in wild birds. But migration pathways bring them in contact with domestic birds, such as chickens, turkeys and ducks. Flu viruses in their urine and feces can cause infections with exceptionally high mortality. that can be passed to domestic flocks. The infection is 100% lethal in domestic birds.

Bronchiolitis: Inflammation of the smallest air passages in the lungs, the bronchioles. The condition is usually caused by viral infection and is more common in children than in adults.

C

C influenza: (*See Type A, B, C influenza*)

CDC: Centers for Disease Control and Prevention. The leading U.S. government health agency that helps to prevent and control infectious and chronic diseases.

Cell culture: Term used in reference to the cultivation and maintenance of cells in a laboratory. The cells are propagated in a growth medium. Cell cultures can be used as a source for producing flu vaccines, which eliminates the need for the age-old technique involving millions of fertilized chicken eggs to produce the annual vaccine doses.

Chemoprophylaxis: Prevention of disease by use of medication.

Common cold: A highly contagious, upper respiratory condition caused by any one of many types of viruses. The common cold is typified by nasal congestion, coughing, sneezing, sore throat, and, in some instances, temporarily losing the ability to taste foods or hear clearly. The common cold also is known as nasopharyngitis and acute coryza. *(See adenovirus, coronavirus, picornavirus, and rhinovirus)*

Coronavirus: A family of viruses that includes those responsible for the common cold.

Cough hygiene: Taking precaution when ill with a respiratory condition to cover a cough with a tissue and to properly dispose of it after use. Coughs should be covered to prevent the spread of infectious viruses to anyone nearby.

Cytokine storm: A potentially lethal immune system response to infection, marked by an abrupt surge in pro-inflammatory proteins known as cytokines—interleukin-1, interleukin-6 and tumor necrosis factor, among others. Scientists theorize a cytokine storm affected young people between the ages of 18 and 40 during the 1918 flu pandemic. The immune system in young adults is very robust and capable of mounting a powerful reaction to an aggressive infection, unleashing an explosive flood of immune system constituents—the cytokine storm. Theory holds that it was such a storm that ravaged the lungs— and caused the deaths—of countless individuals when the highly infectious 1918 influenza virus circulated among human populations.

D

DNA: Deoxyribonucleic acid is the hereditary chemical that makes up our genes. Shaped like a spiraling ladder, DNA is a double-stranded molecule often referred to as a double helix. It is one of two types of hereditary material that encodes genetic information. The other is RNA. Humans' genetic information is encoded in DNA. Genetic information of a flu virus is encoded in RNA. *(See genes and RNA)*

Dog flu: Influenza infection in dogs. The most important strain is H3N8, an equine strain. Scientists first detected it in 2004 after the strain apparently jumped the species barrier from horses to cause a severe flu outbreak in dogs. The strain was found to be highly contagious among canines and quickly spread throughout the United States. The strain now is considered endemic in dogs.

Drift: *(See antigenic drift)*

Drug resistance: A condition in which disease-causing organisms can repel drugs that once destroyed them. Drug resistance occurs when drugs are misused and overused, creating an environment in which the organisms can develop tolerance.

E

Epidemic: Any outbreak of disease in a population that is higher than expected. Epidemiologists use a number of measures before declaring an epidemic. With respect to the flu, the number of hospitalizations and cases of pneumonia are taken into account.

Glossary

Eustachian tubes: The air canals in each ear connecting the middle ear to the throat cavity. The tubes equalize air pressure on both sides of the tympanic membrane (eardrum).

F

Flu: Shortened term for influenza. The flu is a viral illness of the respiratory tract caused by any one of three types of viruses (A, B or C). The flu is highly contagious and can be easily spread person to person. The flu can cause mild to severe illness and is a leading cause of wintertime absenteeism in schools and workplaces. *(See influenza)*

Flumadine: *(See adamantanes and rimantadine)*

G

Genes: The basic fundamental units of heredity, each occupying a precise position on a chromosome. Genes are made up of DNA, and humans have between 20,000 and 25,000 unique genes. A flu virus, by comparison, has only 8 genes. Human genes are carried on chromosomes of which there are 46 (23 donated by each parent at the moment of conception) in the nucleus of each cell. There are approximately 100 trillion cells in the adult human body.

Guillain-Barre syndrome: A rare disorder involving an attack on the nervous system by turncoat constituents of the immune system. It is usually triggered by an acute respiratory or gastrointestinal infection. Nerves become inflamed and weakness occurs. Sometimes the first symptom may be a pins-and-needles—tingling—sensation in the legs. But as it progresses there may be a loss of sensation in the arms, legs and feet. The weakness can spread, causing weakness elsewhere in the body until a patient is nearly paralyzed. Some patients are so severely affected they have to be placed on a respirator. In such extreme instances, Guillain-Barre syndrome is considered life threatening. Even though most people affected by Guillain-Barre syndrome recover, some degree of weakness may persist.

H

H and N: Hemagglutinin and neuraminidase are the two surface proteins on an influenza virus. Hemagglutinin is important because it is necessary for a flu virus to attach itself to a cell in a host's respiratory system. Neuraminidase is an enzyme that is essential for flu viruses to spread throughout the respiratory tract. Once the virus invades the nucleus of a host cell, it then replicates and makes new viruses. Neuraminidase allows the viruses to escape the host cell and infect new cells. Scientists have identified 15 different "H" proteins and 9 different "N" proteins. There are a variety of combinations of these proteins that have been identified. H5N1, an avian strain, is considered a threat because it has never circulated in human populations. Variants of H3N2 circulate seasonally in human populations, triggering seasonal influenza.

Hand hygiene: Frequent hand washing, or at the very least, frequent use of a hand sanitizer to prevent self-infection or passing infections along to others.

Hemagglutinin: *(See H and N)*

Herd immunity: Also called "community immunity," refers to the protection of a small minority of unvaccinated people because the majority in a population has been vaccinated against a contagious illness.

High pathogenicity/low pathogenicity: Terms often used in reference to the infectiousness of microorganisms. The terms have been especially useful in differentiating variants of H5N1 and other avian flu viruses. For example, a variant of H5N1 determined to be of high pathogenicity will produce widespread disease in flocks of domestic birds and carry a high death rate. Low-pathogenic strains, by comparison, are not nearly as lethal because they do not spread as efficiently nor produce high mortality.

Host: The animal (or human) in which a parasite thrives.

I

Immune response: The immune system's reaction to infection, toxins or transplanted organs.

Immune senescence: An aging immune response.

Immune system: The cells, tissues and organs that help the body resist infection and disease by producing antibodies and cells that block the multiplication of an infectious agent.

Inactivated: An inactive agent that has lost its disease-producing capacity.

Influenza: A serious respiratory infection noteworthy for its rapid person-to-person spread. Influenza—the flu—can have limited impact on a community or it can spread rapidly throughout many communities as an epidemic. Either Type A or B influenza viruses are capable of triggering epidemics. Occasionally, when a novel virus *(see antigenic shift)* enters human populations, it can spawn a pandemic, a global outbreak capable of causing massive waves of illness and death. *(See antigenic drift, epidemic, flu, and pandemic)*

L

Low pathogenicity: *(See High pathogenicity/low pathogenicity)*

M

M2-e: A "highly conserved" protein of influenza viruses. By highly conserved it is meant that this protein does not undergo mutations as readily—or as dramatically—as hemagglutinin or neuraminidase, the two proteins that stipple the surface of flu viruses. Scientists are studying the possibility of basing a "universal" flu vaccine on M2-e. A universal vaccine would be one that would be effective against seasonal as well as pandemic strains of influenza.

Mixing vessel: A theory explaining how flu viruses from different species might combine in one animal to produce a novel virus. For example, scientists posit that should swine contract flu viruses from wild birds,

Glossary

pigs may serve as "mixing vessels." Porcine flu viruses, according to the theory, can combine with those from birds to produce a novel pathogen. *(See reassortment)*

Mutation: Any alteration of a gene from its normal sequence of molecular building blocks to a new one. In humans, a mutation might produce a new heritable sequence that leads to a disease that is passed from generation to generation. Small mutations in surface protein genes of seasonal flu viruses allow them to remain infectious year to year. Mutations in flu viruses (or any organism for that matter) are random events and cannot be predicted. The random nature of mutations, according to U.S. government flu researchers, makes it difficult, if not impossible to know, if or when a virus such as H5N1 might acquire the properties needed to spread easily among humans.

N

Neuraminidase: *(See H and N)*

NIAID: National Institute of Allergy and Infectious Diseases, a major division of the National Institutes of Health that conducts and supports basic and applied research into the treatment and cure of allergic and infectious diseases.

O

Oseltamivir: Generic name of the antiviral medication Tamiflu, which is used in the treatment and prevention of both influenza A and influenza B viruses. Oseltamivir is a neuraminidase inhibitor, which means that it prevents the release of new viruses from an infected cell. The drug is marketed by Hoffmann-La Roche. In Japan, it is marketed by Chugai Pharmaceutical Co., which is affiliated with Hoffmann-LaRoche. More than 50 million people have been treated with the drug, the majority in Asia.

Outbreak: A sudden rise in the incidence of a disease.

P

Pandemic: A global outbreak of disease that causes high rates of sickness and death as occurred three times in the 20th century during major flu outbreaks that killed millions of people. Pandemics were documented in 1918, 1957 and 1968. The 1918 pandemic, which occurred at the end of World War I, claimed at least 50 million lives, but possibly millions more. Among Americans, more people died of the flu than were killed in the war.

Parainfluenza virus: A viral infection that causes bronchiolitis (*see bronchiolitis*) and is most often diagnosed in children. Although the name is similar, parainfluenza is not related to the flu and is not caused by any member of the family of viruses that cause the flu.

Pneumococcal pneumonia: A bacterial infection of the lungs which can occur alone or as a secondary infection in someone already affected by the flu. Pneumococcal pneumonia is considered a serious condition because it can spread throughout the lungs, enter the blood stream, middle ear, or nervous system. Vaccines are available to prevent pneumococcal pneumonia.

Prophylactic: Any intervention that prevents or provides protection against a disease or condition. Common prophylactics include vaccines, antibiotics, and antiviral medications.

Q

Quarantine: The period of isolation decreed to control the spread of disease. Before the era of antibiotics, quarantine was one of the few available means of halting the spread of infectious disease. It is still employed today as needed. The list of quarantinable diseases in the U.S. is established by Executive Order of the President, on recommendation of the Secretary of the Department of Health and Human Services, and includes cholera, diphtheria, infectious tuberculosis, plague, smallpox, yellow fever, and viral hemorrhagic fevers (such as Marburg, Ebola, and Congo-Crimean disease). In 2003, SARS (severe acute respiratory syndrome) was added as a quarantinable disease. In 2005 another disease was added to the list, influenza caused by novel or re-emergent influenza viruses that are causing, or have the potential to cause, a pandemic.

R

Reassortment: A rearrangement of genes that emanate from two distinct strains of influenza. The recombination of those genes can produce a novel influenza strain. (*See mixing vessel)*

Relenza: An antiviral medication that must be inhaled as a mist, and is one of two antiviral medications (the other

is Tamiflu) administered to treat both seasonal and avian influenza. Among seasonal flu viruses, Relenza is effective against both Type A and B influenza. Like Tamiflu (oseltamivir), Relenza is a neuraminidase inhibitor. These drugs block the activity of neuraminidase, the flu virus enzyme that allows newly replicated flu viruses to escape the host cell and infect countless other cells in the lungs. When neuraminidase is blocked, the infection process is thwarted. Relenza, a product of GlaxoSmithKline, is also sold under the generic name, Zanamivir.

Respiratory syncytial virus (RSV): A common virus that causes mild respiratory conditions in adults but can cause more serious conditions, such as bronchiolitis, croup, and pneumonia in infants and children.

Rhinovirus: A type of virus that infects the upper respiratory tract and causes the common cold.

Ribonucleic acid (RNA): A nucleic acid molecule similar to DNA but containing ribose rather than deoxyribose. RNA is formed upon a DNA template. RNA tends to mutate at a faster pace than do genes composed of DNA and that is at least one major reason why flu viruses tend to transform themselves so quickly from one season to the next.

Rimantadine: (*See adamantanes and Flumadine)*

S

Seasonal flu: A respiratory illness caused by influenza Type A, B, and

C viruses, which circulate annually worldwide. Flu season, which occurs during fall and winter in the Northern Hemisphere, is preceded by influenza season in the Southern Hemisphere. A key feature of seasonal flu viruses is their capacity to be easily transmitted person to person. Most people have some immunity, but the ever-changing genetic character of the viruses allows them to remain contagious and people are vulnerable to catching the flu throughout their lives. Vaccines are available.

Shift: (*See antigenic shift*)

Spanish flu: A term often used to describe the devastating pandemic of 1918 during which an estimated 50 million people (possibly even twice that number) died worldwide. The term Spanish flu is a misnomer because the influenza outbreak did not begin in Spain. Modern theorists suggest that Spanish health officials were far more open about discussing the widespread contagious illness than were other countries, giving the false impression that the flu began in Spain.

Staphylococcal pneumonia: A bacterial infection that can occur as a secondary condition in people affected by the flu.

Strain: A genetic variant or subtype of a microorganism. For example, influenza Type A varies by strain. The strain is determined by the genetic differences in proteins that make up the flu virus.

Strategic National Stockpile: The stockpile is organized and controlled by the Centers for Disease Control

and Prevention and is designed as a national repository of antibiotics, vaccines, medications, life-support equipment, and medical and surgical supplies. The stockpile is generally referred to as the SNS, and is not simply a single source of supplies but several stored in secret locations throughout the United States. The SNS is deployed during a state of national or regional emergencies, such as the attack on New York's World Trade Center in 2001 and Hurricanes Katrina and Rita in 2005. In the event of a major flu pandemic, the SNS would be deployed.

Streptococcal pneumonia: A bacterial infection that can occur as a secondary condition in people debilitated by the flu. Streptococcal pneumonia is commonly referred to as Pneumococcal pneumonia. There is a vaccine.

Symmetrel: (*See adamantanes*)

T

Tamiflu: The highly potent antiviral used to treat both seasonal and avian influenza. (*See oseltamivir*)

Type A, B, and C influenza: Pathogens that belong to the family of orthomyxoviruses. Scientists have defined three distinct types. Type A can trigger seasonal flu as well as seasonal epidemics. All three major pandemics in the 20th century and the major pandemic of 1889 were caused by Type A flu strains. Waterfowl are considered the natural reservoir of Type A flu viruses. H5N1, an avian flu strain, is a Type A virus. Type B influenza occurs only in humans, but like Type A, can be associated with epidemics. The annual flu vaccine provides protection against two Type A strains and one Type B. Type C is a much milder form of influenza and manifests as an illness that is very similar to the common cold. Type C protection is not included in annual flu vaccines.

U

Universal vaccine: A flu vaccine that can be administered against any seasonal strain as well as serve as a preventive against any emergent pandemic strain. Scientists who are working on various types of universal vaccines say a universal flu immunization might also require periodic boosters to help people maintain sufficient antibody protection.

V

Vaccine: A preparation consisting of a weakened or killed pathogen, such as a bacterium or virus. Only a mere snippet of a pathogen is required to create a vaccine. Vaccines do not function like medicines. Instead, they stimulate the immune system to fend off infection by producing antibodies; it is antibodies that fight the infection. The immune system produces antibodies in response to antigens, which are the surface proteins on the bacterium or virus used to create a vaccine. Antibodies are so precise that should someone be exposed to influenza, the immune system of a vaccinated person is already primed to fight the infection.

W

W curve: When scientists produced graphs illustrating mortality during the 1918 pandemic, they discovered an unexpected W-shaped pattern, which reflected spikes in the number of deaths of very specific age groups. For example, the first "arm" of the W reflects a high number of deaths among infants during that outbreak and a dip in mortality at ages 5 through 14. The next peak in deaths was unexpected, and involved people roughly between the ages of 18 and 40 who usually are considered to be in robust health and able to fight off a severe infection. However, scientists now theorize that young adults died as a result of their own immune systems' aggressiveness. In an effort to destroy the virus, the body unleashed a flood of antibodies and other immune system components that proved lethal *(see cytokine storm)*. The other arm in the W reflected an increased number of deaths among the very old, people in their late 70s and older.

WHO: World Health Organization, an agency of the United Nations which plays a vital role in a variety of global health concerns, particularly in identifying and studying various strains of influenza that are chosen for each year's vaccine.

Z

Zanamivir: Generic name for Relenza, an antiviral medication prescribed to treat cases of influenza. It is also used as a flu prophylactic when administered within the first 48 hours of infection. (*See Relenza*)

Index

Index

Index

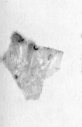